# The Golfer's Nutrition Caddy

## Your guide to staying strong, focused, and energized from tee off to final putt!

**Anita Duwel**

**Certified in Holistic Nutrition and Health**

# Dedication

*To all golfers:*

*may this guide fuel your passion, support your health,*

*and empower you to play with energy, focus, and vitality*

*both on and off the course.*

---

*To my beautiful granddaughter Maty:*

*whose fun-loving spirit reminds me every day*

*to embrace life with wonder, curiosity, and awe.*

*And to my wonderful family*

*for your unwavering support and encouragement*

*both on and off the course.*

# Disclaimer

The information in *The Golfer's Nutrition Caddy* is for general educational purposes and not a substitute for medical advice, diagnosis, or treatment. While this book highlights how nutrition and hydration can support better performance on the course, it's not intended to treat or cure any condition.

Before making changes to your diet, fitness, hydration, or supplement routine, check in with your doctor — especially if you have health conditions or take medication.

Every golfer is different. This book shares evidence-informed strategies, but your choices should be guided by your unique needs and medical history.

The author and publisher are not liable for any loss or injury resulting from how you use this information. By reading this book, you agree to take full responsibility for your health and performance.

And hey, even the best players check in with their caddies. When in doubt, talk to your doc before you tee off on a new routine.

# Table of Contents

# Hole 1

# Welcome!

Welcome to "The Golfer's Nutrition Caddy!"

I'm so very happy to have you here!

One thing I want to be clear about is that this is not a book that will tell you what you can and cannot eat. I believe that a healthy balance is what we should all be striving for.

You can still have a burger with fries or ice cream!

What's important is that you eat well most of the time. A perfect formula is that 80% of the time, you make healthy choices and 20% of the time, you can have an indulgence or two.

If you have a poor diet, this book will guide you through the changes you can make and why it is important to both your golf game and your health.

I strongly suggest that you make small changes at a time. Trying to revamp everything, all at once, will only make it difficult to maintain, and you will most likely revert back to your old ways.

**So, your mantra should be one step at a time.**

If you eat pretty well, then this book can help guide you on what to eat and when to eat in order to play your best.

Golf is a game that, in addition to skill, requires physical and mental stamina from the moment you tee off until you drop that last putt.

And, if you want to have the energy you need to play your best golf, then start thinking about what you feed your body!

**Does this sound familiar?**

You're at the 13th hole and you find your energy levels are dipping, you're starting to lose focus, and your swing just doesn't feel right.

You're feeling some frustration and not scoring as well as you should be.

And, you really can't figure out why.

The answer may just be in your nutrition!

The right foods can keep your energy levels up, help you concentrate, and even speed up your recovery after a tough round.

In this book, you'll learn about the importance of macronutrients (carbohydrates (carbs), proteins, fats) and micronutrients (vitamins and minerals).

We'll chat about hydration (extremely important) and provide practical tips to help you stay hydrated on the course.

Plus, we'll discuss what types of foods to eat and when.

We even have a chapter with lots of easy, tasty recipes to help you fuel up before a round, keep your energy levels up during play, and recover well afterwards.

If you play competitive golf or travel for golf, we have you covered!

And, for those of you who may have some special dietary considerations, we'll address them as well.

Whether you're a weekend warrior or a seasoned competitor, "The Golfer's Nutrition Caddy" will provide you with the information you need to make smart decisions about your nutrition that can help take your golf game to the next level.

At the next Hole, we'll spend a little time discussing the gut-brain connection (amazing and powerful) and how it can improve both your mental and physical performance on the course.

# Hole 2

# First Tee Fundamentals

## The Gut-Brain Connection

As you are aware, when playing golf, you need to be focused, be able to make good decisions, and have your stress under control. Not so easy sometimes!

Well, believe it or not, your gut might just be the unexpected MVP of your game!

The gut, also known as the second brain, communicates directly with your brain, which affects everything from mental clarity and mood to physical endurance.

This is known as the gut-brain connection.

And, this gut-brain partnership needs to be working well together for you to physically and mentally play your best.

Imagine your gut and brain as two teammates constantly passing notes. This communication network, known as the gut-brain connection, relies on the vagus nerve for communication back and forth and a network of neurons in your gut (enteric nervous system).

What's very interesting is that 80-90% of the neurons in the vagus nerve carry information from the gut to the brain.

Wow! This means the signals that are coming from the gut have a huge influence on your mood, behavior, and even cognitive processes.

Therefore, your gut is not just about digestion.

If your gut is healthy, you're more likely to stay focused, keep your cool, and feel strong throughout your game.

But if things are off balance?

You might find yourself feeling drained and unable to concentrate.

So, in a sport that demands both mental strength and physical endurance, it becomes important that you keep your gut in check.

Let's look at a few ways this "second brain" impacts your game.

## 1. Stress and Emotional Balance

**Gut's Role**: Around 95% of your body's serotonin (the feel-good hormone) is produced in your gut!

When things are good with you, you're more likely to stay calm, positive, and resilient. But if things are out of balance, you might find yourself feeling frustrated or stressed.

**Golf Impact**: Staying calm under pressure is huge for golf. A steady mental state keeps you swinging smoothly. Taking care of your gut health may just be your secret to handling high-pressure shots and situations and staying cool and calm on the course.

## 2. Concentration and Mental Clarity

**Gut's Role**: Your gut microbiome (the bustling community of bacteria in your gut) has an effect on your brain's performance.

These microbes help regulate memory, focus, and clarity. Therefore, a healthy gut can sharpen thinking and decision-making.

**Golf Impact**: Clear, focused thinking is essential for making decisions related to the type of shot, distances, club selection, course conditions, etc.

Keeping your gut in top shape may help improve your concentration, giving you an edge when it matters most.

### 3. Physical Stamina and Recovery

**Gut's Role**: Your gut doesn't just help you digest food … it's where you absorb nutrients that power your body, strengthen your immune system, and keep you energized.

**Golf Impact**: From the first tee to the 18th green, endurance is everything. A gut that's in great shape means steady energy levels and quicker recovery.

### 4. Managing Nerves and Pre-Game Jitters

**Gut's Role**: We've all felt those "butterflies" in our stomach before something big … that's your gut and brain chatting about stress!

When your gut health is balanced, it can keep your nerves in check, helping you feel grounded.

**Golf Impact**: Whether you're on the first tee or facing a tournament-deciding putt, a calm, centered feeling can make all the difference.

A balanced gut can play a subtle but crucial role in managing nerves.

**Note:** Having some "butterflies" in your stomach can be good. However, too much stress can jeopardize your playing ability.

Here are 5 gut-friendly tips that can help *Boost Your Gut Health.*

## 1. Focus on Fiber-Rich Foods

**Impact:** Fiber is like food for your gut bacteria, keeping them happy and helping with smooth digestion. Load up on fiber from fruits, veggies, and whole grains to keep that gut microbiome in top form.

**Golf Benefit:** A balanced microbiome can help you stay calm, focused, and energized all the way through a long game.

## 2. Stay Hydrated

**Impact:** Water isn't just for hydration; it keeps your digestion running smoothly and helps support gut-brain communication. Proper hydration also regulates mood and cognitive function.

**Golf Benefit:** Good hydration helps with focus and endurance, keeping you mentally and physically sharp.

## 3. Add Probiotics and Prebiotics

**Impact:** Probiotics (found in foods like yogurt and kefir) boost your gut health, while prebiotics (found in foods like bananas and garlic) feed these good bacteria.

**Golf Benefit:** A stronger gut microbiome can lead to better focus, less stress, and improved physical strength.

## 4. Manage Stress Off the Green

**Impact:** Chronic stress can be tough on the gut-brain connection, so practicing relaxation techniques … like yoga, breathing exercises, or meditation … can really help.

**Golf Benefit:** A calm, steady mind, supported by a healthy gut, allows you to handle stress and play with confidence.

## 5. Prioritize Quality Sleep

**Impact:** Sleep is critical; as it's the time when the body can repair and restore, especially for your gut and brain.

**Golf Benefit:** With good sleep on your side, you can arrive at the course well-rested, mentally sharp, and physically prepared.

### Summary

The gut-brain connection may not be the first thing you think of when improving your golf game, but it's a powerful … and often overlooked … part of the puzzle.

By adding gut-friendly habits into your routine, you're boosting not only your physical health but also your mental clarity and resilience.

Just as you would practice your different shots or study the course, taking care of your gut health is an investment in your game that pays off in focus, calmness, and energy.

At the next hole, we'll take a look at nutrition. Specifically, macronutrients (carbohydrates, proteins, and fats) and their role in your gut health and your ability to perform at your best on the golf course.

# Hole 3
# Fairway Foods
# Understanding Golf Nutrition
# (Macronutrients)

Welcome to your nutritional tee-off!

Just like mastering your swing and staying focused on the green, understanding nutrition basics can make a really big difference in your game.

Nutrition is more than just fuel … it's about getting the right balance of energy and nutrients to support physical stamina, mental clarity, and recovery.

We're going to begin by talking about the three macronutrients: carbohydrates, proteins, and fats.

They are the powerhouses that give you what you need to stay sharp and energized.

### Macronutrients: The Power Trio

Think of macronutrients as the A-team of nutrients that keep you performing at your best.

- **Carbohydrates**: These are your body's go-to for fuel, providing the energy you need to power through long rounds and maintain focus throughout your game.

- **Proteins**: They are needed for muscle maintenance and recovery. They repair and strengthen your muscles.

- **Fats**: They are a steady, slow-burn fuel that provides lasting energy and supports heart and brain health.

EACH macronutrient plays a crucial role.

Your goal is to get the right balance of them so that your performance will be where you want it to be.

## Carbohydrates (Carbs): The Caddies of Your Energy

Are you in the camp that thinks all carbs are bad for you?

I'm very happy to tell you that not all carbs are evil. In fact, some are ESSENTIAL!

Carbs received a bad rap when highly processed, refined foods, such as candy, cookies, white bread, and sugary cereals flooded supermarket shelves. These items are loaded with empty calories and have absolutely NO nutritional value.

However, carbs such as fruits, veggies, and whole grains are EXCELLENT carbs, and they come loaded with fiber, protein, B vitamins, and numerous other nutrients that make a real difference to your health.

These are the carbs you should be happily adding to your plate!

For golfers, understanding the role of carbohydrates is critical.

But beware! Not all carbs play the game the same way.

**Complex vs. Simple Carbs**

- **Complex Carbs**: Found in foods like whole grains, vegetables, and legumes. They break down slowly, providing a steady release of energy without a crash.

Complex carbs support endurance and mental focus, perfect for a long round of golf.

- **Simple Carbs**: Simple carbohydrates, such as sugars and refined grains, provide a quick burst of energy that fades quickly.

  This roller coaster of energy levels can lead to fatigue, affecting your performance, especially in the later stages of the game. Not what you want on the golf course!

By choosing complex carbohydrates for your meals, you ensure that your body is fueled and ready to go.

**Example:** Before a game, a bowl of oatmeal with berries provides long-lasting energy, keeping you sharp and ready through all 18 holes. (more recipes at Hole 14)

## Next on the Tee: Proteins, Your Muscle Repair and Maintenance Crew

Proteins work diligently behind the scenes, much like the grounds crew of a beautifully maintained golf course.

They are essential as their job is to repair and maintain the muscular system that powers every aspect of your game.

Every swing you make, every step you take, and even the simple act of carrying or pushing your golf bag stresses your muscles, causing micro-tears that need timely repair.

Protein steps in to repair those tiny tears, preventing muscle soreness and injury while also building stronger muscle fibers for future performances.

Following are some of the key muscles that are involved in your golf game, and eating enough protein will help keep them healthy and strong.

- **Core Muscles**: These stabilize and help transfer power from your lower to upper body.

- **Shoulders and Arms**: Essential for swing control and range of motion.

- **Hip:** Pivotal in creating and controlling the rotational force. They also help maintain balance and stability.

- **Back**: Involved in the rotational movements required for a powerful swing.

- **Legs**: Provide stability and power during the swing

A protein-rich snack post-round, like a smoothie or chicken wrap, helps with muscle repair, reduces soreness, and keeps you strong.

Since you have muscle from head to toe, you want to be sure to include protein in your daily diet.

Protein also plays an important role in producing key hormones and enzymes that keep your body balanced and energized.

Here's a basic look at how these "behind-the-scenes" players work to support your game:

## Hormones: Manage Stress, Energy, and Focus

- **Focus and Energy:** Proteins help produce hormones like adrenaline and noradrenaline, which sharpen your focus under pressure, and testosterone, which supports muscle strength and stamina.

- **Mood and Sleep Regulators:** Tryptophan, an amino acid found in protein-rich foods like turkey, eggs, and dairy, is essential for producing serotonin and melatonin.

  - ‣ **Serotonin:** Regulates mood and concentration, helping you stay calm and focused.

  - ‣ **Melatonin:** Great for sleep and recovery, which translates to a good day of golf.

## Enzymes: Your Body's Nutrient Breakdown Squad

Enzymes, powered by proteins, act as your body's "Nutrient Breakdown Squad," helping transform the carbs, fats, and proteins you eat into usable energy.

Think of them as your body's hidden maestros:

- **Amylases:** The carb connoisseurs. Found in saliva and the pancreas, they begin breaking down complex carbs into simple sugars for quick energy as soon as you start eating.

- **Lipases**: Your fat breakdown experts. These enzymes turn fats into fatty acids and glycerol, which provide the long-lasting energy needed to maintain stamina.

- **Proteases**: The muscle allies. Its role is to break protein down into amino acids, which will support muscle repair and growth.

So, the next time you pack for the course, consider your protein intake as a necessity.

Whether you're enjoying a protein-packed smoothie, a handful of nuts, or a hearty chicken wrap, fueling up on these powerhouse nutrients ensures that you are ready to play your best.

Protein isn't just part of the meal; it's part of your strategy to outlast and outperform your competitors or finish a game feeling strong!

## Next up Fats: The Long-Game Strategists

Embrace the fats! Healthy fats are an underrated powerhouse in a golfer's diet.

Research has shown that healthy fats are a critical component of a balanced diet; for sustained energy, cellular function, nutrient absorption, and overall health.

They're like your long-game strategists … providing slow-release energy that lasts for hours, supporting endurance, mental clarity, and even joint health.

While their benefits might not be immediately apparent, healthy fats provide a slow-releasing energy source that powers you through all 18 holes.

This makes them indispensable for a sport that can last four hours or more.

**Types of Fats and Their Benefits**

Not all fats are created equal. Here's a breakdown of the different types of fats and how they benefit your game:

- **Monounsaturated Fats**: Found in foods like avocados, nuts, and olive oil, these fats support heart health and reduce inflammation, helping maintain endurance and overall well-being on the course.

- **Polyunsaturated Fats**: This category includes omega-3 and omega-6 fatty acids; essential fats the body can't produce on its own.

  Omega-3 and omega-6 fatty acids, abundant in sources like fish, nuts, and seeds, are especially beneficial for cognitive health and reducing inflammation.

- **Saturated Fats**: While it's best to consume these in moderation, saturated fats (found in meat, butter, and coconut oil) provide a quick energy source and support hormone production, essential for overall health and stamina.

## Avoiding Trans Fats

One type of fat you'll want to avoid is **trans fats**.

Trans fats are found in many processed and fried foods. They increase inflammation, negatively affect heart health, and can lead to sluggishness … all things you want to avoid on the course.

- **Common Sources**: Packaged baked goods, fried foods, margarine, pre-packaged snacks, and some microwave popcorn.

- **Tip for Avoiding Trans Fats**: Check food labels for "partially hydrogenated oils" or "hydrogenated oils," which indicate trans fats.

- **Opt for whole foods and snacks** made with healthy fats, like nuts or fresh avocado, instead.

## The Anti-Inflammatory Aces

Omega-3 fatty acids, a type of polyunsaturated fat found in fish oil, flaxseeds, and walnuts, are particularly valuable for golfers.

They help control inflammation, which can intensify during long games and rigorous practice sessions.

These fats reduce muscle soreness and protect joints, both of which are crucial for golfers facing repetitive swings and long days on the course.

If you minimize inflammation, you can help prevent injuries and maintain flexibility for a smooth, pain-free swing.

**Pro tip:** Aim to include omega-3-rich foods like salmon, chia seeds, or walnuts a few times a week. A serving of fatty fish or a handful of nuts is a great addition to your diet for overall joint and heart health.

### Beyond Sustained Energy

Incorporating healthy fats from avocados, nuts, seeds, and fatty fish, such as salmon, into your diet can help regulate blood sugar levels, reduce the risk of heart disease and type 2 diabetes, and enhance brain function.

These fats also serve as powerful anti-inflammatories and may lower the risk of conditions such as arthritis, cancer, and Alzheimer's disease.

Omega-3 fats (fish, flax seeds, chia seeds, walnuts) are important for optimum nerve, brain, and heart function.

## Fats are Essential in Absorbing Key Vitamins

Vitamins A, D, E, and K are fat-soluble, meaning they need fats for proper absorption.

These vitamins are vital for bone health, immunity, and antioxidant support, which is key to maintaining strength and stamina on the course.

Without adequate healthy fats, your body can't effectively absorb these vitamins, which could lead to deficiencies that could impact both your health and your golf performance.

For example, insufficient vitamin D and calcium absorption due to low fat intake can lead to weaker bones, increasing the risk of fractures … a significant concern for any golfer.

## Smart Integration

Incorporating healthy fats into your diet isn't about going overboard with any and all types of fat.

It's about choosing the right types in the right amounts.

Like choosing the right club for a particular shot, it's about adding the right type of fats in moderation.

Snack on a handful of almonds or walnuts, add a few slices of avocado to your salad, or drizzle some olive oil on your veggies.

Healthy fats are continuously at work, optimizing your body's performance both on and off the course.

So the next time you prepare for a day on the links, remember: fats are as essential to your game as a club is for a well-executed putt or a perfectly timed swing.

But, beware, as fat is high in calories. It is the most energy-dense of the three macronutrients, coming in at 9 calories per gram vs 4 calories per gram for both protein and carbohydrates.

Therefore, check your portion sizes!

A portion size of healthy fats can vary based on dietary needs and individual health goals, but a general guideline is:

- **Nuts and seeds:** About 1 ounce (a small handful), which is roughly 28 grams or ¼ cup.

- **Nut butter:** Approximately 1 to 2 tbsp.

- **Avocado:** About ¼ to ½ of a medium avocado.

- **Olive oil:** 1 tbsp, which is about 15 milliliters.

- **Fatty fish (like salmon):** A serving is typically around 3 to 4 ounces (about the size of a deck of cards).

**Example Day of Meals for a Golfer** (more ideas and recipes can be found at Hole 14)

To help you visualize how to incorporate macronutrients throughout your day, here's a sample meal plan to fuel a round.

| Sample Meal Plan | |
| --- | --- |
| Breakfast | Oatmeal with berries and a boiled egg (complex carbs, fiber, protein) |
| Mid AM Snack | Greek yogurt with a handful of almonds (protein, healthy fats) |
| Lunch | Grilled chicken wrap with a whole-wheat tortilla, avocado, and mixed greens (protein, healthy fats, fiber) |
| On Course Snack | Banana and a handful of almonds (carbs, magnesium, healthy fats) |
| Dinner | Salmon with quinoa and roasted veggies (protein, omega-3s, complex carbs, antioxidants) |

## Summary

A balanced mix of carbohydrates, proteins, and healthy fats isn't just solid nutrition … it's your secret weapon for a winning game.

I hope this has provided you with a clearer understanding and inspired you to consider making incremental adjustments to your diet.

These changes can help elevate your game and ensure you perform at your best.

At the next hole, we'll delve into the world of micronutrients and explore how they can help take your performance to the next level.

# Hole 4

# Micronutrients

# Essential Extras For Optimal Performance

Now that you're getting the hang of macronutrients, let's dive into the smaller but very important players in your nutrition game: micronutrients.

These vitamins and minerals don't provide direct energy like carbs or fats, but they're essential for muscle function, mental clarity, and endurance.

### Key Micronutrients for All Golfers

**Iron:** The Heavy Hitter for Energy.

Iron is a powerhouse for energy. It helps make hemoglobin, which transports oxygen from your lungs to your muscles and brain … vital for stamina and concentration.

- **Where can you get iron from?** Lean meats, poultry, spinach, and iron-fortified cereals can be combined with vitamin C-rich foods, (such as bell peppers or oranges) to boost nutrient absorption.

- **Who Benefits Most?** Women, particularly those of menstruating age, need more iron to avoid fatigue, while both younger and older golfers benefit from iron to support endurance and muscle health.

**B Vitamins:** The Energy and Focus Boosters.

B vitamins are key to converting the food you eat into usable energy (ATP), helping you maintain focus and mood during a round.

They also support brain health, which means improved decision-making and mental endurance … perfect for us golfers who need to stay focused.

- **Where can you get your B vitamins from?** Whole grains, lean meats, eggs, legumes, and leafy greens.

- **Who Benefits Most?** All golfers benefit from B vitamins, especially if they need steady energy and mental sharpness. Older adults particularly benefit as B-vitamin absorption can decrease with age.

**Calcium and Vitamin D:** The Dynamic Duo for Bones.

This duo is all about strong bones and muscles. Calcium builds and maintains bone strength, while Vitamin D helps with calcium absorption and supports muscle contractions.

For us golfers, they're needed for stability and power.

- **Where can you find calcium and vitamin D?** Dairy products, fortified plant milks, leafy greens, and fatty fish such as salmon.

  And, you can get it naturally from sunlight. All you need is 15 minutes out in the sun.

  You can also take a D3 supplement. Speak to your doctor about this.

- **Who Benefits Most?** Women, particularly post-menopause, need to focus on calcium and Vitamin D to prevent bone density loss.

  Older men benefit from Vitamin D for bone and muscle health, as well as testosterone support.

**NOTE:** Vitamin D needs healthy fats to be absorbed effectively. Pair it with fats such as avocado or olive oil for maximum benefit.

**Magnesium:** The Muscle and Recovery Mineral.

Magnesium supports muscle function, helps prevent cramps, may reduce inflammation, and aids in relaxation … perfect for golfers who need endurance on the course and effective recovery afterwards.

- **Where can you find magnesium?** Leafy greens, nuts, seeds, and whole grains.

- **Who Benefits Most?** Everyone! Younger athletes use magnesium for muscle function and energy, while older golfers benefit from its role in bone health, heart health, and sleep quality.

**Pro Tip:** Magnesium taken in the evening can improve relaxation and recovery.

**Omega-3 Fatty Acids:** Joint and Heart Health for All Golfers.

Omega-3 fatty acids are needed as they provide anti-inflammatory benefits that help keep your joints flexible and reduce pain.

I've learned that taking care of my knees is non-negotiable. After multiple surgeries and with some arthritis setting in, they tend to get inflamed and sore, especially when I push them too hard. That's why omega-3 fatty acids have become a big part of my health routine.

Making sure to get enough omega-3s has made a difference. It's not a miracle cure, but I've noticed that when I consistently include omega-3s in my diet, my knees feel less stiff and achy after a game of golf.

Omega-3s also support heart and brain health, improving endurance and mental clarity … key for consistent performance and focus.

- **Where can you find omega-3 fatty acids?**

  ▸ Fatty fish, such as salmon, sardines, and mackerel.

  ▸ Plant-based sources such as flaxseeds, chia seeds, and walnuts.

  ▸ Different oils, such as olive oil, flaxseed oil, and avocado oil.

- **Who Benefits Most?** All golfers will benefit from omega-3s. Their joint-supporting and heart-health benefits are important when it comes to completing a round of golf with sustained resilience.

**Pro Tip:** Aim for two servings of fatty fish per week, or consider a fish oil supplement if you're not getting enough omega-3s through your diet.

**The Nutritional Scorecard:** Putting Micronutrients to Work.

By incorporating these key micronutrients into your daily intake, you're optimizing:

- **Endurance:** Sustained energy and mental clarity.

- **Muscle Support:** Strong muscles and reduced cramping.

- **Injury Prevention:** Solid bone health and reduced injury risk.

It's a good idea to track your micronutrient intake so that you can identify areas where you may need a boost.

A balanced approach, with a variety of nutrient-dense foods, keeps you at the top of your game on and off the course.

**Action Steps for Optimal Micronutrient Intake**

For your next round, try adding these nutrient-dense options:

- **Pre-game snack:** Greek yogurt with berries (for calcium and antioxidants).

- **On-course fuel:** A banana or orange for potassium and a handful of nuts for magnesium.

- **Post-game recovery:** Grilled salmon with quinoa and spinach to replenish iron, omega-3s, and magnesium.

With this strategic approach, you'll set yourself up for a stronger, more resilient game.

**Next up:** Hydration and electrolytes, because staying hydrated is as crucial as fueling your body with the right nutrients.

# Hole 5

# Hydration

## The Foundation of Peak Performance

### Why Hydration Gets Its Own Spotlight

You've probably heard the advice to "stay hydrated" more times than you can count, along with the usual mention of electrolytes.

And maybe you sip water throughout your round and add some electrolytes for good measure.

But the big question is, "Are you hydrating enough?"

My guess is … probably not.

Staying hydrated is key to maintaining your game and your health, but it's also essential to boosting it.

Fact. If you are not hydrated enough, you cannot play at your full potential.

Think of water as the greenskeeper for your body. It keeps everything lush, playable, and free from the "sand traps" of fatigue, poor focus, and muscles that just aren't performing.

**Did you know that** our bodies are about 60% water? And the brain? About 73% water!

Those numbers show hydration is crucial for overall health and peak cognitive function.

Even a tiny 2% drop in hydration can be a problem for your brain! WOW!

And that becomes a problem for your golf game.

If you find that your focus starts to slip, it could be that you're dehydrated and your sodium and electrolytes are low.

So, to keep your mind sharp and your body humming, ensure you're sipping enough water throughout the day!

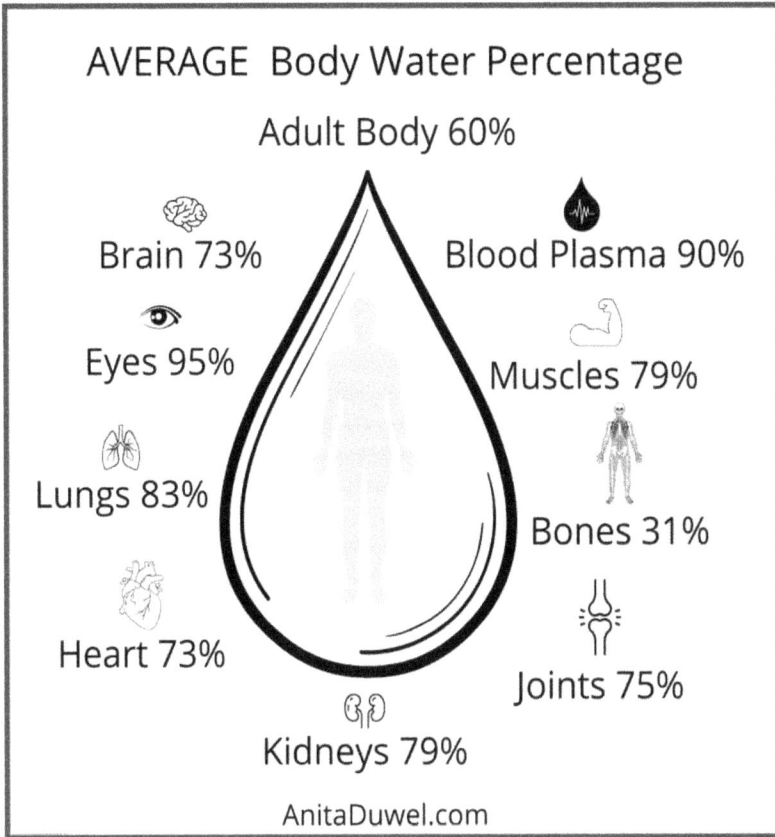

AVERAGE Body Water Percentage
Adult Body 60%
Brain 73%
Blood Plasma 90%
Eyes 95%
Muscles 79%
Lungs 83%
Bones 31%
Heart 73%
Joints 75%
Kidneys 79%
AnitaDuwel.com

This image showing the water composition of different parts of our body might make you reconsider just how essential it is to stay hydrated.

Stay hydrated, and you stay sharp!

As golfers, concentration, coordination, and endurance must be at their best through hours of play. Hydration isn't just a nice-to-have; **it's non-negotiable.**

**The Critical Role of Hydration in Golf**

Picture this:

You're playing your round of golf, it's hot, and you are sweating. You did drink your water ... heck, you had a one-liter bottle that is now empty, and you are quite proud of yourself for drinking all of it.

Maybe you're even thinking of a nice cold drink at the 19th hole.

At the end of the round, you're discussing with your playing partners how you seemed to lose steam and focus over the last 5 or 6 holes that you played. Maybe they did too.

Well, a good reason for that may just be that you did not drink enough water.

During a regular round of golf, you can lose anywhere from 2 to 4 liters of water through sweat alone. You heard that right!

So that one liter that you did drink was not nearly enough to keep you hydrated which, in turn, could be the reason for your loss of energy and focus on the back nine.

Sweating is your body's way of cooling itself down (that's a good thing) ... the problem is that you are also losing valuable fluids and electrolytes. Not good!

Is drinking water enough?

No.

On warm days, not only is drinking enough water important but so is the addition of electrolytes as they replace the loss of sodium and potassium. (More on electrolytes a little further on)

On a hot, humid day, the amount of water loss you experience climbs even higher, making dehydration a real risk if you're not actively hydrating.

When you are not hydrating enough, things start to slip (and so will your game):

- **Mental focus:** Dehydration can reduce cognitive function, affecting decision-making and accuracy.

- **Physical energy:** You might feel fatigue, muscle cramps, or coordination issues … none of which are great for your swing!

- **Overall stamina:** Even mild dehydration can throw off your game, turning a potentially great round into a struggle.

Did you know that water's role goes beyond satisfying thirst?

- It regulates body temperature.

- Maintains blood pressure.

- Supports muscle and joint function.

Even more reason to stay hydrated both on and off the course!

The big question is, "How much do I need to drink?"

**General Guidelines**: The amount of water a golfer should drink during a round depends on different factors, such as the weather, size, age, fitness level, and how much they sweat.

As a rule of thumb:

- A simple calculation to help you determine your ideal DAILY intake is to drink half of your body weight in fluid ounces or multiply your body weight by two-thirds.

  For example, if you weigh in at 150 pounds, then your goal would be to drink 75 to 100 ounces (2.2-3 liters) of water **for the day.** (Very important that you create a habit of drinking water throughout the day and not just when on the course)

- On the course, you want to be sipping water throughout the 18 holes.

  Your goal would be to drink about 4-6 ounces of water every 15 minutes, depending on the temperature and how much you sweat.

  Try taking a sip or two after every shot.

**Hot Weather Adjustments:** If you're playing in hot, humid weather, it becomes crucial to increase your hydration:

- Try drinking **20 ounces (about .6 liter) of water every three holes** to stay ahead of dehydration.

**Personal Note:** My Garmin watch does more than track my steps … it also monitors my hydration! On extremely hot days, my water loss has reached 100 ounces (around 3 liters); on a typical hot day, it's closer to 64 ounces (about 2 liters).

And when I don't drink enough, I feel the difference … I am not at my best. My focus is lost and my energy is low. There have been times when I felt lightheaded, which is not a good feeling! Plus, I become at risk of heat stroke!

This is a perfect example of why staying on top of hydration is so important … especially during those long rounds under the sun!

**Make sure to start your round hydrated.**

If you're only drinking water when you're thirsty, it's already too late.

Thirst is your body's way of saying, "Hey, I'm low on water!" This means that your hydration strategy should kick in BEFORE you feel thirsty.

A smart approach is to start hydrating a few hours **before** tee-off.

Aim for about 16-20 ounces (500-600 ml) of water two to three hours before you start. This pre-hydration phase sets up a hydrated baseline for the day and will help your body absorb the water for peak benefit.

**The Power of Electrolytes (Just as important as water)**

Let's talk electrolytes … those little minerals like sodium, potassium, and magnesium that make all the difference in hydration.

In addition to losing water, you also lose these very important minerals.

When you only replenish with plain water, you risk diluting your blood sodium levels, which can lead to headaches, confusion, and, in severe cases, even seizures (known as hyponatremia).

What do these minerals do?

- Sodium helps with water retention.

- Potassium supports muscle function.

- Magnesium helps prevent cramps.

Adding electrolytes to your water, especially on hot or high-intensity days, can make a big difference … and not just for your performance, but for your health, too!

Therefore, make sure to add electrolytes to your water or you can make your own electrolyte drink.

Commercial sports drinks can be effective, but beware, as they are often loaded with sugar and artificial colors, so check the label first.

For example, a 20-ounce bottle of a regular sports drink can contain 35 grams of sugar, while its sugar free option has none. Always do your homework on any electrolyte drinks you choose to ensure they're high quality.

## DIY Electrolyte Boost: Homemade Recipe

Here's a very easy-to-make electrolyte drink that will help you stay hydrated, replace lost electrolytes, and has a bit of sweetness to keep your energy and your body well-hydrated on the course.

### Ingredients

- 1 liter of water

- Juice of ½ lemon or lime (adds flavor and has vitamin C)

- ¼ tbsp of Himalayan pink salt (for sodium and trace minerals)

- 1-2 tbsp of honey or maple syrup (for a natural energy boost)

- A pinch of baking soda (optional; adds a bit more sodium to help with hydration)

**Instructions**

1. Put all the ingredients in a jug and mix until the honey or syrup and salt are completely dissolved.

2. Pour it into a thermos and drink it throughout the day.

This drink provides the right amounts of sodium, potassium, and magnesium to support hydration and muscle function … perfect for a long round of golf!

Plus, it doesn't contain any artificial colors or sugars often found in store-bought sports drinks.

**Another great hydrator is coconut water**

Coconut water is a fantastic hydration choice for golfers, and here's why:

- **Natural Electrolytes**: Packed with potassium, sodium, magnesium, and calcium, coconut water helps maintain hydration and muscle function.

- **Hydrating and Refreshing**: High water content and natural electrolytes make it ideal for rehydrating before a long game.

- **Low-Calorie and Natural**: Unlike many sports drinks, coconut water is low in calories and sugars, so you get the nutrients without the unnecessary additives.

- **Natural and Minimally Processed:** Coconut water is a natural beverage with minimal processing. It doesn't contain artificial additives, colors, or preservatives commonly found in many commercial sports drinks.

- **Rich in Potassium**: Potassium is a vital electrolyte that helps prevent muscle cramps and supports proper muscle function. Coconut water contains more potassium than many sports drinks, making it an excellent choice for athletes.

- **Antioxidant Properties**: Coconut water contains antioxidants that can help reduce muscle fatigue and improve recovery.

**Following is a great pregame recipe with coconut water.**

**Pregame Coconut Water Smoothie**

This smoothie is a tasty way to fuel up with carbs, protein, healthy fats, and hydration.

**Ingredients**

- 1 cup fresh spinach

- 1 banana, sliced

- ½ cup Greek yogurt

- 1 tbsp almond butter

- ½ cup coconut water

- Ice cubes (optional for a thicker consistency)

**Instructions**

1. Add all ingredients to a blender.

2. Blend on high until smooth and creamy.

3. Pour into a glass and enjoy!

## Spotting Dehydration Before It Hits Your Game

Knowing the signs of dehydration can help you catch it before it has too much of an impact on your performance. Common symptoms include:

- Feeling thirsty or having a dry mouth

- Fatigue or dizziness

- Infrequent bathroom trips or dark-colored urine

- Headaches or light-headedness

Step up your fluid intake immediately if you notice any of these signs. Sip on water or your homemade electrolyte drink to help restore your hydration quickly.

## Hydration as Part of Your Golf Strategy

Think of hydration as part of your game plan, just like choosing the right club or gauging the wind. Regular, proactive hydration ... before, during, and after play ... keeps your performance at its peak and helps you avoid the dreaded effects of dehydration.

Before heading out, ensure you're well-hydrated, and keep your water bottle as handy as your favorite putter.

With each hole, take a moment to drink, ensuring hydration throughout the day.

This disciplined approach to hydration will support your body's needs and can dramatically improve your focus, energy levels, and overall golf performance.

**IMPORTANT: Hydration is a Gradual Process**

You can't just chug your daily intake in one sitting and expect to be fully hydrated and game-ready. Staying consistently hydrated each day is the real key to optimal performance.

If this is not a habit you have, try to make an effort to take a sip after every shot or between shots as you walk to your ball.

Connecting your sips to your shots will help make the water habit stick!

"Water is the most neglected nutrient in your diet, but one of the most vital."-Julia Child.

Now that you know the types of foods to eat and are hydrated, you're ready to take on the next step: pregame prep.

At Hole 6, we're teeing up the ultimate pregame fuel!

Discover exactly what to eat and drink before you step onto the course so you're primed for all-day energy and peak performance.

# Hole 6

# Prime Your Game

## Your Pre-Round Nutrition Playbook

Every great game doesn't just start with a good warm-up ... it starts with smart fueling.

Think of your body as your most reliable club in the bag, one that needs the perfect mix of fuel to hit those long shots and keep your focus sharp all the way to the 18th hole.

Just like you wouldn't tee off with a putter, you wouldn't start your round on an empty tank ... or worse, filled with the wrong kinds of snacks.

In this chapter, we're diving into the art and science of pregame fueling.

You'll learn how to master meal timing, what to eat, and even when to eat so you're powered up without feeling weighed down. Getting your nutrition right can transform your game, whether your tee time is early in the morning or late in the day.

We'll explore foods that give you steady energy without the dreaded crash (goodbye, midgame meltdowns!) and share tips for keeping things tasty and simple ... because fueling up doesn't have to be bland.

Let's approach your nutritional prep with the same focus you bring to your game.

**Menu for a Powerful Tee-Off (3-4 Hours Before Game Time)**

Alright, golfers, it's time to fuel up *before* you hit the course!

Think of your body like a high-performance sports car. You wouldn't dream of hitting the racetrack on an empty tank, right?

It's the same with golf. A well-balanced meal before your round can make all the difference in your focus and endurance.

So, what's on the menu?

## Balanced Breakfast

Start with a combo of complex carbs, lean protein, and healthy fats. (Remember how essential these macronutrients are from Hole 3?)

How about a hearty bowl of oatmeal topped with fresh berries and a drizzle of honey, paired with a couple of scrambled eggs?

Or, if you're more into smoothies, blend up some spinach, banana, Greek yogurt, and almond butter.

Both options will keep you full and focused.

For some great, easy recipes, head to Hole 14.

## Why a Balanced Breakfast Wins

Let's break down how a balanced breakfast helps your game:

- **Jumpstarts Your Metabolism**: Golf requires hours of sustained energy. Starting your day with a balanced meal improves your metabolism, ensuring that the food you have consumed is converted to needed energy.

- **Provides Steady Energy**: Golf rounds are long and require CONSISTENT energy. A mix of carbs, proteins, and fats provides a slow release of energy, preventing mid-round fatigue.

- **Improves Focus and Concentration**: Precision is key in golf. A stable blood sugar level from a balanced breakfast supports mental clarity, so you'll be sharp for every shot.

- **Enhances Physical Performance**: Walking the course and swinging repeatedly requires endurance. A balanced breakfast fuels your muscles, giving you the strength and stamina you need.

- **Supports Weight Management**: A good breakfast helps curb hunger and prevents overeating, which supports a healthy weight … key for mobility and balance on the course.

- **Promotes Overall Health**: Eating well regularly keeps you healthy and less likely to be sidelined by fatigue or illness, so you're always ready to play.

Each benefit of a balanced breakfast supports aspects of your golf performance, from sustained energy and improved concentration to physical endurance.

Go to Hole 14 for some breakfast recipes that will provide you with the nutrients that you need.

**When You Need an Energy-Boosting Snack**

If your tee time is later in the morning, you might need a little energy boost to hold you over.

Think apple slices with almond butter, a handful of trail mix, or a yogurt parfait with granola.

The goal? Stick to whole, unprocessed foods that give you energy without the crash and avoid sugary or heavy foods that might slow you down or leave you feeling sluggish.

**Quick Bites Before the First Swing**

Sometimes, the morning gets away from you.

Maybe you hit the snooze button too many times or got caught up in pregame nerves.

No worries! If you're heading to the course and realize you need a quick energy fix, try one of these quick and easy bites:

- **Energy Bars**: Go for bars with natural ingredients and a good balance of protein and carbs. Avoid the sugary options that can lead to a crash.

- **Fruit**: Bananas, apples, or a handful of berries are easy to pack and provide quick energy.

- **Nuts and Seeds**: A small handful of almonds, walnuts, or pumpkin seeds gives you healthy fats and protein.

- **Yogurt**: A small container of Greek yogurt with granola or honey is satisfying and energizing.

Remember, the goal is to fuel up without feeling full and weighed down.

These quick bites will steady your energy levels so you can focus on your game, not your grumbling stomach.

**Timing Your Meals for Game-Day Energy**

Timing is everything in golf, and the same goes for your meals.

To optimize your energy levels and avoid any mid-game slumps, it's important that you time your meals and balance your intake.

- **3-4 Hours Before**: Have a substantial meal, like the balanced breakfast mentioned earlier. This gives your body time to digest and convert food into usable energy.

- **1-2 Hours Before**: Time for a small, energy-boosting snack. Apple with peanut butter or a small yogurt with granola will do wonders without making you feel sluggish.

- **30 Minutes Before**: If you're feeling hungry, grab a light snack, like a piece of fruit or an energy bar, for a last-minute boost. The key is to keep it light and easy to digest.

Recipes can be found on Hole 14.

By spacing out your meals and snacks, you're giving your body a steady stream of fuel, so you're ready to perform at your best from the first swing to the last putt.

Think of it like putting premium fuel in your car; your body deserves the best to perform at its best!

**Hydrate, Hydrate, Hydrate!**

Food is only part of the equation … hydration is equally important.

You won't be at your best if you're not properly hydrated by game time!

Start your hydration strategy early. Aim to drink at least 16 ounces of water when you wake up.

Then, about 30 minutes before game time, do a hydration check. This is a great time to have some water with electrolytes or a glass of coconut water for an extra electrolyte boost.

## How to Do a Hydration Check

A hydration check is a simple way to ensure you're adequately hydrated before hitting the course. Here are a few easy ways to gauge your hydration:

- **Monitor Urine Color**: The color of your urine is a good indicator. If it's light yellow or nearly clear, you're likely hydrated. Dark yellow or amber means you should drink more water.

- **Skin Elasticity Test**: Gently pinch the skin on the back of your hand. If it snaps back quickly, you're well-hydrated. If it takes a moment to return to normal, it might be a sign you need more water.

- **Check for Dry Mouth or Thirst**: If you feel thirsty or notice a dry mouth, it's already a sign of mild dehydration. Make sure to drink water before you start.

- **Energy Levels**: Low energy can also be a hydration red flag. If you feel sluggish or have low energy before your game, try drinking a glass of water with electrolytes to see if it boosts your alertness.

And remember hydration isn't just for game day; it's a habit that should stay with you even when you're off the course.

Staying consistently hydrated day-to-day ensures you're always ready to perform, no matter when you tee off.

So, next time you're gearing up for a game, remember this chapter and fuel up like the golf pro you are!

At the next hole, we'll explore fairway nutrition, breaking down the best snacks and strategies to keep your energy high and your focus sharp.

Let's ensure you're fueled and ready to finish as strong as you start!

# Hole 7

# Power Up the Fairway

## Maintain Focus and Energy with Smart Snacking

Alright, you've teed off, and you're making your way down the fairway. How do you keep your energy up without filling your body with junk?

It's snack time!

But not just any snacks … we're talking about power-packed bites that keep your swing strong and steady, round after round.

**Nuts and Dried Fruit:** Small but Mighty.

Think almonds, walnuts, pistachios … small but mighty snacks that are perfect for a steady energy boost. A handful provides protein, healthy fats, and fiber for slow, steady fuel.

Pair them with a few dried apricots or raisins for natural sugars that give you a quick lift without the crash.

**Bananas:** Nature's Energy Bar.

A good old-fashioned banana. Packed with potassium, it helps fend off muscle cramps, making it perfect as a mid-game snack.

Plus, it comes in its own biodegradable wrapper! Eat one at the turn, and you're good to go.

**DIY Energy Balls:** Custom Fuel, Just for You.

Try whipping up a batch of energy balls. Mix oats, peanut butter, honey, flax seeds, and a sprinkle of chocolate chips. Roll into bite-sized balls, chill in the fridge, and toss a few in your bag. (See recipe at Hole 14)

They're like tiny bursts of energy that taste awesome and help keep your muscles happy! For variety, you can add chopped dried fruit or shredded coconut.

**Energy Bars:** Choose Wisely.

Beware! Not all energy bars are created equal! Choose bars made from whole ingredients (think nuts, seeds, and oats) and low in added sugar to avoid a post-snack crash.

Look for around 10-15 grams of protein to keep you satisfied. Keep a couple in your bag for a quick energy boost.

If you would like to make your own, check out the recipe at Hole 14.

**Veggie Sticks and Hummus Packets:** Crunchy and Refreshing.

For something fresh, pack pre-cut veggie sticks such as carrots, bell peppers, or cucumbers and pair them with a small pack of hummus.

This combo gives you hydration, fiber, and a bit of protein without weighing you down. And they're refreshing on a hot day!

I often bring chopped peppers and cucumbers ... very refreshing.

Here are some more easy snack ideas:

- **Apple Slices and Peanut Butter:** Preslice apples and pack a small peanut butter container for dipping.

- **Cheese Sticks:** String cheese or individual portions of cheeses like cheddar or gouda are great for calcium and protein.

- **Hard-Boiled Eggs:** Peel them ahead of time for a quick, protein-rich snack.

- **Trail Mix:** Make your own with a mixture of dried fruits, nuts, and seeds, perhaps with dark chocolate. Recipe at Hole 14.

- **Fresh Fruit:** Bananas, oranges, and grapes are easy to handle and provide natural energy-rich sugars. Watermelon is my favorite, especially on hot days.

- **Roasted Chickpeas:** Season and roast chickpeas for a crunchy, protein-packed snack. Recipe at Hole 14.

- **Rice Cakes and Almond Butter:** A light snack that's easy to pack and customize with toppings like almond butter or a slice of turkey.

- **Turkey Jerky:** Opt for low-sodium, natural varieties of jerky for a lean protein fix.

- **Edamame:** Precooked and shelled edamame is rich in protein and fiber and easy to eat on the go.

- **Mini Sandwiches:** Whole grain bread with fillings like turkey, spinach, and a slice of cheese can be made into small, easy-to-eat sandwiches.

You want your snacks to be light yet sustaining so that you can enjoy your game without feeling weighed down or hungry.

**Bonus Snack Tips for Golfers**

- **Timing is Key**: Don't wait to grab a snack until you're feeling low on energy. Try to take a few bites every few holes to keep your energy steady and avoid a crash.

- **Choose Portable, Easy-to-Eat Snacks**: Go for snacks that can handle a bit of warm weather and are simple to eat between holes.

  Whole fruits, energy balls, and nuts are perfect on-the-go options that require minimal prep and keep you fueled without any fuss. Pack them in small, reusable containers to stay organized.

- **Keep It Balanced**: Try to include a mix of carbs, protein, and healthy fats in your snacks. Carbs give quick energy, protein keeps you full and your muscles like it, and fats give longer-lasting fuel.

- **Pack Smart:** If you don't have an insulated pocket in your golf bag, you can use a small insulated bag for items that need to stay cool, and make sure to keep your snacks easily accessible so you're not digging around trying to find things.

By stocking your golf bag with smart, balanced snacks and keeping these tips in mind, you'll keep your energy and focus up, setting yourself up for a good game from start to finish!

**Don't forget your hydration!**

Be sure to have enough water with electrolytes or coconut water to keep you hydrated throughout the round.

Small sips after every shot are a great way to help you stay hydrated. See Hole 6 for more info on hydration.

At the next hole, you will find a guide on how you can organize your snacks for maximum performance.

# Hole 8

# Guidelines For On-Course Snacking

## Fuel Your Round With The Right Foods At The Right Time

The timing of what and when you eat on the golf course is important for maintaining steady energy levels and focus throughout your game.

Following is a sample guideline to help you manage your snacking.

### Early Holes (1-6)

Your goal is to consume fast-digesting carbohydrates that provide a quick energy boost. Make sure they are not full of added sugars or highly processed foods.

The suggestions below will give you the fuel you need without weighing you down.

**Snack Options:**

- **Fresh fruit** (like an apple or banana) contains natural sugars for immediate energy and hydration.

- **Granola bar**: A compact option that's easy to eat between shots. Look for one with whole grains and minimal added sugars.

- **Trail mix**: A mix of dried fruit, nuts, and seeds provides quick carbs along with a bit of healthy fat to keep you going. (recipe at Hole 14)

- **Watermelon** is high in water content (about 90%), making it great for hydration early in your round. It provides quick, easily digestible carbs from natural sugars, which offer a fast energy boost without weighing you down. It's also refreshing and helps keep you cool, especially in warmer weather.

## Middle Holes (7-12)

As you move through the middle part of your round, your energy needs to stay stable to keep your game sharp. A mix of carbs, protein, and healthy fats will maintain your energy without causing crashes.

**Snack Options:**

- **Mixed nuts and dried fruit**: Carbs from the fruit, protein and healthy fats from the nuts for endurance.

- **Peanut butter and banana/jelly sandwich on whole grain bread:** Whole grain bread provides slow-digesting carbs, while the peanut butter adds protein and healthy fats, and the banana/jelly offers a quick carb boost.

- **Apple slices with almond or peanut butter:** The apple provides quick-release carbs, while the nut butter adds protein and healthy fats.

- **Hard-boiled eggs with a handful of mixed nuts:** The eggs provide protein, while the mixed nuts offer a combination of protein, fat, and carbs for sustained energy.

- **Greek yogurt with chia seeds and berries**: Greek yogurt offers protein, the berries provide antioxidants and carbs, and chia seeds add healthy fats.

- **Bell peppers with hummus or some nuts:** Bell peppers are packed with vitamin C, antioxidants, and fibre. They provide hydration, a little crunch, and steady energy without being heavy. Pair them with hummus or a small handful of nuts for added protein and healthy fats.

**Final Holes (13-18)**

During these final holes, you want to maintain steady energy and hydration while starting to focus on muscle recovery.

Your body is working hard at this stage, so a slight increase in protein is key.

**Snack Options:**

- **Turkey and avocado wrap**: Lean protein from the turkey and healthy fats from the avocado, wrapped up in a light tortilla for easy, balanced fueling. Tofu can replace the turkey to make it a vegan option.

- **Cheese stick with whole grain crackers**: A small, easy-to-digest snack with protein and fiber to keep you full and satisfied.

- **Hummus with veggie sticks**: A plant-based option with fiber, protein, and healthy fats that'll keep your energy up and muscles supported.

Maintaining steady energy during your round is crucial, but post-game nutrition is just as important for recovery and replenishing lost nutrients.

At Hole 9, we will explore the essential steps for refueling after the game to prepare you for your next round.

# Hole 9

# 19th Hole Recovery

# Post-Game Nutrition

## Repair and Recharge: Foods that Mend Muscles and Mood

After a day of chasing pars, birdies, or bogeys, dealing with bunkers and the rough, and overcoming wayward shots, your body's more than ready to take a break.

Just as you make sure to put away your clubs, gloves, range finder, etc, you should also take care of your post-game nutrition.

This is your chance to help your body repair and recharge.

Think of your muscles like caddies ... they've been lugging you all over the course, and now they need some TLC.

Protein is your go-to here. Lean chicken, turkey, fish, vegetarian protein, or a plant-based protein shake can do the trick. These foods help repair muscle fibres, ensuring that you're ready for your next tee-off.

But what about your mood and mental focus? Foods rich in omega-3 fatty acids, like salmon or flax seeds, can help keep your mental game strong.

Protein is the repair crew, and healthy fat is the sports psychologist. Together, they keep your muscles and brain happy and healthy.

### Quenching Your Thirst Post-Round

You've been out there, under the sun, swinging and walking. Chances are, you may be dehydrated.

Hydration isn't just about drinking during the game. After your last putt, what you sip can set the stage for recovery and your next performance.

Water is the undisputed champion here. And if you are having difficulty ensuring you get enough of it, maybe you need to jazz it up a bit.

You can add some orange or cucumber to your water. Not only does it refresh, but it also adds a hint of electrolytes back into the body.

Or, have some electrolytes (homemade, store-bought or coconut water) to help you hydrate.

### Relaxing Meals to End Your Golf Day

Ending the day should feel as good as sinking a long putt.

This is your time to unwind and enjoy a meal that satisfies both the stomach and the soul. Helping you to relax and replenish.

Imagine sitting back with a plate of grilled salmon, sweet potato, and a heaping of greens. It's not just delicious; it's a nutritional powerhouse, providing a balanced mix of protein, carbs, and fats to help your body recover and prepare for the next challenge.

Or maybe you're in the mood for something simple like a pasta dish with lean beef and plenty of veggies in a light tomato sauce. It's comforting, filling, and keeps those recovery bases covered.

In the spirit of the 19th hole, it's about relaxation and enjoyment. So choose foods that you not only benefit from but also genuinely enjoy.

Remember, the 19th hole is as much about celebrating the day's play as it is about setting you up for success in future rounds.

Check out the recipes at Hole 14 for some post-game meals.

Cheers to good food, good health, and great golf!

While post-game nutrition helps replenish your body, mindful eating takes your overall health to the next level by developing a deeper connection with your food.

At Hole 10 we'll explore mindful eating … ensuring you're not just feeding your game but also nurturing a balanced and intentional relationship with food, on and off the course.

# Hole 10

# Conscious Consumption

# Mindful Eating for Golfers

Welcome to the Zen zone of your golf game ... your plate!

Just like a smooth swing depends on mindful movements, improving your nutrition comes down to paying close attention to when, what, and how you eat ... mindful eating.

### Mindful Eating and How it Helps Golfers

Mindful eating isn't just about slowing down how you eat; it's also about experiencing food with all your senses: taste, touch, smell, sight.

Picture this: You're standing on the green, the sun is setting, and you've just unpacked a snack. Instead of gobbling it down, you take a moment to really look at it, smell it, and appreciate its textures. You take a bite and savor the taste ... you are present and in the moment.

This isn't crazy; it's strategy.

Why? Because golf also requires awareness. The more in tune you are with your body's hunger signals and feelings of satiety, the better you can fuel your rounds without overeating or undereating.

It's about eating with intention. Choosing snacks that sustain energy, not just quick and convenient ones. And as we all know, quick and convenient means high sugar and crashes ... leaving us with no energy in the last part of our game.

Think of mindful eating as your secret weapon for sustained focus and energy, so important for those back-nine battles.

Plus, it teaches you to be present and in the now ... whether it's when you're eating or when you're taking a shot.

## Techniques to Master Mindful Eating On and Off the Course

Ready to master mindful eating? Start with these quick tips:

1. **Engage Your Senses:** Before you eat, take a deep breath and engage your senses. How does the food look, feel, and smell? This will help your brain register the meal ahead and get your digestive system ready.

2. **Eat Slowly:** Take small bites, chew thoroughly, and put your food or fork down between bites. Slowing down helps you digest better and recognize when you're full, preventing that sluggish feeling that can wreck your rhythm.

3. **Check-In With Yourself:** Ask yourself: Am I really hungry, or am I just bored or stressed? Recognizing real hunger cues will help you avoid eating unnecessary snacks that can lead to a mid-round crash.

And in general, this will help with weight management and overall health.

4. **Plan Your Meals:** Just as you plan your game strategy, plan your eating strategy. Align your meals and snacks with your tee times to ensure you're fueled and ready to go.

   For some of you, this may mean having an online/written schedule with a menu planned out.

   This will help you stay away from a hotdog and soda at the turn!

   See Hole 7 for ideas and a sample of what to eat over the 18 holes.

- **Make Smart Choices for Better Performance:** The food you choose is just as important as how you eat it. That means opting for foods that boost concentration and help sustain energy.

Complex carbohydrates like whole grains, proteins like chicken, fish, legumes, tofu, and fats from sources like avocados and nuts are super choices. They keep your energy levels steady, allowing you to maintain focus and power through an entire round.

Imagine you're lining up for a putt on the 18th green and if you make it, you have played the best game of your life. Because you have fueled well and stayed hydrated, your focus and energy are good, and you feel in control. You make the putt and celebrate with your foursome. Congratulations, what an awesome feeling!

If you had played on sugary snacks and hadn't paid attention to hydration, you may not have had the energy or focus to have been in that position on the 18th hole.

By being mindful about what and when you eat, you're setting yourself up for better rounds and a healthier, more aware lifestyle.

It's all about making every bite count just as much as every putt. So, here's to eating mindfully and lowering those scores, one conscious bite at a time!

Just as practicing mindful eating can keep you steady at the tee box and on the green, it can also guide you when you're far from your usual kitchen.

At the next hole, we'll take these principles on the road so you can fuel yourself just as effectively, no matter where your travels lead.

# Hole 11

## Smart Eats When You're On the Road

Travel days can be quite challenging for maintaining good nutrition habits. It used to be the norm that road trips were synonymous with munching on processed snacks like chips, cookies, and other packaged treats. (at least when I was younger.)

I now eat better on the road, and it's amazing how much of a difference it makes!

The key is preparation.

Remember, maintaining your golf game on the road isn't just about keeping your swing in shape. It's also about fueling the machine that makes those swings!

By planning ahead and making smart food choices, you can ensure that your nutrition stays on par, no matter where your travels take you.

## Packing the Perfect Golf Trip Pantry

When you're packing up your clubs, shoes, and other gear needed for your golf trip, don't forget something that is just as important: your nutrition.

Stock up on non-perishable, nutrient-dense options like mixed nuts, low-sugar protein bars, dried fruit, trail mix, and whole-grain crackers. Small packets of almond butter or hummus are great, protein-packed snacks.

If you have a cooler with you, add in items such as cut-up veggies, yogurt, hard-boiled eggs, and some chicken, turkey, or tofu wraps.

This is one lesson I have learned over the years … to pack my own snacks; otherwise, I was eating way too much junk food bought at roadside stops.

And all it did was leave me feeling bloated and, quite frankly, not good at all.

Now, when I travel, I munch on the snacks I bring with me … making the trip that much more enjoyable! Bonus: I feel better, too!

## Dining Out Tips and Tricks

Eating out doesn't have to throw your healthy habits off-course.

**You can:**

- Choose grilled instead of fried.

- Ask for sauces and dressings on the side.

- Customize your meal. Most places are happy to swap out fries for a salad or vegetables.

- Check out the menu online before you go. That way, when you show up hungry at the restaurant, you will know what you want and will not end up ordering something that is greasy and heavy.

- Think about when you eat. A heavy meal right before tee time can weigh you down, while a lighter, balanced meal can help you stay energized and focused.

- The same goes for at night. You don't want to be eating a heavy meal before bedtime.

- And don't forget to stay hydrated. Keep that water bottle close to you at all times. A clear head and a steady swing go hand in hand.

Being well-prepared with the right nutrition while traveling does more than just keep you physically fit. It plays a crucial role in maintaining mental sharpness and focus, the key to playing good golf!

Now that you've got your on-the-go nutrition locked in, it's time to bring those skills to the big event.

At Hole 12, we'll focus on tournament-day strategies, ensuring you show up at the tee with steady energy and ready to tackle the course.

# Hole 12

# Championship Chow

# Eating Right to Endure the Long Haul of Tournament Play

It's the first day of your tournament ... not just any day ... it's 'the' day. The greens are pristine, the fairways are lush, and the stakes are high. You're excited and nervous.

You're feeling the pressure. Now, some pressure is good and feeling a bit nervous can be good as well. However, it's important to keep your nerves and stress under control.

This is where your nutritional game can make or break your golf game.

If your nutrition is off and you're fueling up on sugary or processed foods, it'll be tough to stay calm, finish the tournament strong, and perform your best.

Plus, a dehydrated body will definitely not help you.

In fact, you will begin to lose focus and concentration starting on the first day. And then struggle through the remaining days.

So, how do you fuel your body so that you can stay strong physically and mentally over the whole tournament?

## Breakfast of Champions

Start your day like a champ. Think of your breakfast as the foundation that will keep you strong throughout the day.

A good analogy here is that of your home. You need a solid foundation to keep your home stable and strong. If that foundation was built on something wobbly, it wouldn't hold up.

That goes for you as well … if you don't start your day off strong, you won't hold up either.

A breakfast of champions would consist of a mix of complex carbs, protein, and healthy fats.

A bowl of oatmeal topped with nuts and berries or eggs with whole-grain toast and avocado will keep your energy levels steady and your mind sharp.

## Timing is Everything

When you're playing multiple rounds, it's important to keep track of your meal and snack schedule so you don't run out of energy.

Don't let more than three hours go by without eating something. Make sure to keep snacks like energy bars, a banana, or a peanut butter sandwich in your bag. These quick bites can help prevent hunger and keep your focus on the game, not your growling stomach.

For a guide on what to eat during your game, refer back to Holes 7 and 8.

## Hydration: Your Secret Weapon

Staying hydrated is essential for every golfer. Dehydration is sneaky and can creep up on you, making it harder to concentrate and draining your energy, just like a water hazard swallowing up your ball.

Start drinking fluids when you wake up and keep sipping throughout the day. In fact, you should be hydrated long before the tournament weekend to ensure proper hydration.

Water is great, but on long, hot, sweaty days, a sports drink can help replace lost electrolytes. You can buy one, or you can make your own. (see recipe at Hole 5) Coconut water is also great for hydration.

Think of it as your built-in cooling system, keeping you steady and focused.

**What to Eat Between Two Rounds on the Same Day**

If you're playing 36 holes on the same day, your goal is to refuel efficiently without feeling sluggish.

**Your meal should:**

- Contain protein for muscle support.

- Have complex carbs for sustained energy.

- Be easy to digest to avoid bloating or fatigue.

- Be hydrating to prevent dehydration and cramping.

**For example:**

- Turkey and avocado wrap on whole-grain tortilla with a handful of nuts and a banana.

- Grilled chicken with quinoa or brown rice and roasted vegetables.

- Peanut butter and banana sandwich on whole grain bread and some Greek yogurt.

- Salmon and sweet potato bowl with steamed greens.

- Protein smoothie (banana, almond butter, protein powder, and coconut water).

- Hard-boiled eggs with hummus and whole-grain crackers.

**What to Avoid:**

- Heavy, greasy, or fried foods which can cause sluggishness.

- High-sugar snacks that can lead to crashes.

- Sugary sodas or excessive caffeine.

- Overeating as large portions are hard to digest.

And don't forget to hydrate!

## What to Eat Between Tournament Days (Overnight Recovery Meals)

If you're playing in a multi-day tournament, your focus should be on muscle recovery, glycogen replenishment, and reducing inflammation while ensuring your body is fueled for the next day.

### Key Nutrients to Focus On:

- Protein (for muscle repair) such as salmon, chicken, tofu, eggs.

- Complex carbs (for glycogen replenishment) such as brown rice, quinoa, oats, sweet potatoes.

- Healthy fats (to reduce inflammation) such as avocados, nuts, olive oil.

- Antioxidants (to reduce muscle soreness) such as berries, spinach, turmeric.

- Hydration (to prevent fatigue) such as water, electrolyte drinks, herbal teas.

**Best Dinner Options Between Tournament Days:**

- Grilled salmon with quinoa and roasted asparagus.

- Chicken/tofu stir-fry with brown rice and mixed veggies.

- Baked sweet potato with black beans, avocado, and Greek yogurt.

- Omelet with spinach, mushrooms, and feta cheese and whole grain toast.

- Lentil soup with whole-grain bread and a side of steamed veggies.

- Grilled steak with roasted Brussels sprouts and mashed sweet potatoes.

**Before Bed:**

- Tart cherry juice (has melatonin for better sleep and reduces inflammation).

- Greek yogurt with berries and honey (protein and antioxidants).

- Almond butter on whole grain toast (slow-digesting carbs and healthy fats for steady overnight energy).

- Cottage cheese with almonds (casein protein for overnight muscle repair).

The ideal timing between dinner and a bedtime meal/snack for a golfer (or any athlete for that matter) depends on digestion, energy needs, and sleep quality.

### Here's a general guideline:

- 2 to 3 hours before bed: Have your dinner to allow for proper digestion.

- 30 to 60 minutes before bed: Have a small, nutrient-dense bedtime snack to support overnight recovery and prevent waking up hungry.

**NOTE:** Hold off on any alcoholic drinks, as they will impede the recovery process.

**It's not the time to experiment!**

Stick to foods your body knows and loves. The last thing you need is an upset stomach throwing off your game.

Think of your go-to meals as your culinary caddie … they know exactly what you need and when you need it.

**Tournament is over and its time to celebrate**

Whether you're celebrating a big win or just taking in the lessons of the day, you've earned the right to celebrate.

Make sure to keep it balanced. Enjoy a good meal and a glass of something special; just don't let that glass turn into the whole bottle, as too much alcohol can sabotage your recovery.

Incorporating these nutritional strategies into your tournament play can have a big impact on your performance, your stamina, and your recovery.

Time your meals right, stay hydrated, and stick with what works.

Here's to keeping your energy high and your shots on target!

Now that you've got your tournament strategy figured out, let's explore how to handle those unique dietary needs that might come into play.

At the next Hole, we'll look at special considerations … like food allergies or certain eating styles … so you can stay on top of your game no matter what's on your plate.

# Hole 13

# Special Dietary Considerations

### Tailoring the Menu: Gluten-Free, Vegan, and Dairy-Free

When it comes to eating well, one size doesn't fit all.

If you're gluten-free, vegan, or dairy-free, tailoring your meals is a lot like getting custom-fitted clubs. It helps you play at your best.

Let's look at how you can make simple tweaks so that your nutrition works with you and not against you.

- **Gluten-free?**

  Don't just rely on bread substitutes. Whole, naturally gluten-free options like quinoa or sweet potatoes can keep you fueled with the energy you need without the unwanted inflammation.

- **Vegan?**

  You can get your protein from nuts, seeds, and legumes. They are easily added to salads or homemade energy bars, helping you maintain focus and steady energy when you need it.

- **Dairy-free?**

  Switch to calcium-fortified alternatives such as almond milk or coconut yogurt. You'll get the nutrients you need, minus the lactose that can leave you feeling off your game.

**Adapting Classic Recipes for All Dietary Needs**

Who says you have to give up your favorite fairway foods? All you have to do is adapt them.

Love a good burger? Try a juicy, grilled Portobello mushroom cap or a hearty black bean patty. Both pack flavor and are friendly for most diets. In fact, I enjoy those more than a regular burger as they are so flavorful!

Prep your trail mix the way you want it. Mix up your nuts, seeds, and dried fruits to suit your needs, and throw in some dark chocolate chips for a bit of sweetness.

With a little creativity and planning, you can enjoy delicious, healthy meals that keep your body in golf-ready shape.

Following are three adapted recipes that are perfect for a day on the golf course. They're easy to prepare, portable, and will keep your energy levels up from the first hole to the last.

### Quinoa Salad Jars

### Ingredients

- 1 cup quinoa (cooked according to package instructions and cooled)
- ½ cup cherry tomatoes, halved
- ½ cucumber, diced
- ¼ cup red onion, finely chopped
- ¼ cup feta cheese, crumbled (optional)
- 2 tbsp olive oil
- 1 tbsp lemon juice
- Salt and pepper to taste
- Fresh parsley or basil, chopped.

## Instructions

1. Whisk together the olive oil, lemon juice, salt, and pepper in a small bowl to make your dressing.

2. In a large mixing bowl, combine the cooked quinoa (should be cooled), cherry tomatoes, cucumber, and red onion.

3. Pour the dressing over the quinoa mixture and gently toss to coat.

4. Spoon the quinoa mixture into portable jars. If using feta, sprinkle it on top, along with the fresh herbs.

5. Seal the jars and keep them refrigerated until you're ready to eat.

6. When it's time to eat, give the jar a shake and then enjoy!

## Gluten-Free Turkey and Spinach Wraps

## Ingredients

- Gluten-free tortillas
- Turkey breast slices or legumes or tofu

- Baby spinach leaves

- Sliced avocado

- Mustard or hummus for spreading

- Salt and pepper to taste

**Instructions**

1. Lay a gluten-free tortilla flat on a piece of aluminum foil.

2. Spread a thin layer of mustard or hummus over the tortilla.

3. Add a layer of turkey breast slices, followed by a handful of baby spinach and a few slices of avocado.

4. Season with salt and pepper.

5. Carefully roll the tortilla into a wrap, tucking in the edges as you roll. Wrap tightly in aluminum foil for easy transport and eating on the go.

**Almond Butter and Banana Energy Bites**

**Ingredients**

- 1 cup old-fashioned oats (ensure they're gluten-free)

- ½ cup almond butter

- ¼ cup honey or maple syrup

- ½ cup mashed ripe banana

- ½ tbsp cinnamon

- ¼ cup mini chocolate chips (ensure they're gluten-free)

## Instructions

1. In a large bowl, mix the oats, almond butter, honey/maple syrup, mashed banana, and cinnamon until well combined.

2. Fold in the mini chocolate chips.

3. Scoop the mixture and roll it into bite-sized balls. Place them on a baking sheet lined with parchment paper.

4. Refrigerate the energy bites for at least an hour to set, then transfer them to an airtight container.

5. Keep refrigerated until ready to pack for the golf course.

These recipes are not only gluten-free but also packed with nutrients to help sustain energy, making them perfect for a day of golf.

Here's a recipe for homemade vegan energy bars that are perfect for anyone needing a quick, nutritious boost.

**Vegan Energy Bars**

**Ingredients**

- 1 cup rolled oats (ensure they're gluten-free if necessary)
- ½ cup raw almonds or walnuts, chopped
- ½ cup dried cranberries or raisins
- ¼ cup pumpkin seeds
- ¼ cup sunflower seeds
- ¼ cup flaxseed meal
- ½ cup unsweetened shredded coconut
- ¼ cup chia seeds
- 1 tbsp cinnamon
- ¼ tbsp salt
- ½ cup almond butter or peanut butter
- ⅓ cup maple syrup or agave syrup
- 1 tbsp vanilla extract

## Instructions

### 1. Prep the Dry Ingredients

In a large mixing bowl, combine the oats, chopped nuts, dried fruit, pumpkin seeds, sunflower seeds, flaxseed meal, shredded coconut, chia seeds, cinnamon, and salt. Stir until everything is well mixed.

### 2. Mix Wet Ingredients

In a small saucepan over low heat, gently warm the almond butter and maple syrup/agave syrup until smooth and easily pourable. Remove from heat and stir in the vanilla extract.

### 3. Combine and Press

Pour the almond butter mixture over the dry ingredients. Mix well with a spoon or your hands until all the dry ingredients are evenly coated.

Line an 8x8 inch baking dish with parchment paper, allowing some overhang for easy removal. Transfer the mixture to the baking dish. Press firmly into the pan until the mixture is compact and even. This is crucial to ensure the bars hold together.

## 4. Chill and Set

Refrigerate the mixture for at least 2 hours or until firm. This helps the bars set and makes them easier to cut.

## 5. Cut and Serve

Lift the bars out of the pan using the overhanging parchment paper. Transfer to a cutting board and slice into bars or squares.

Store the bars in an airtight container in the refrigerator for up to a week or freeze them for longer storage.

These vegan energy bars are not only delicious but also incredibly versatile. Feel free to swap in different nuts, seeds, or dried fruits based on your preferences or what you have on hand. They're perfect for a pre-workout snack, a midday energy boost, or even a quick breakfast on the go!

Now that we've talked about personalizing your meals to meet your needs, you can adjust any recipe that you find.

At the next hole, we'll roll out more golfer-friendly dishes that keep you well-fueled and are easily tweakable so you can stay on top of your game.

# Hole 14
# Easy Yummy Recipes
# To Fuel You For Great Golf

This is your nutrition caddy packed with recipes that will keep your energy up from the first tee to the 18th green.

From breakfasts that start you off strong to snacks that keep you steady and dinners that help you wind down, every meal plays a role in your performance.

If need be, the following recipes can be easily adapted to meet your dietary needs.

## BREAKFASTS TO START YOUR DAY RIGHT

### The Early Bird Smoothie

Kick off your day with a blend that's both energizing and easy to digest. It's quick, it's portable, and it gets your engine running without weighing you down.

## Ingredients

- 1 ripe banana

- 1 scoop of your preferred protein powder

- 1 cup unsweetened almond milk

- 1 tbsp chia seeds

- A handful of fresh spinach.

## Instructions

1. Place all ingredients in a blender.

2. Blend on high until smooth.

3. Pour into a glass and enjoy a quick, nutrient-packed breakfast to start your day.

## Par-Fect Protein Pancakes

## Ingredients

- 1 cup oat flour

- 1 tbsp baking powder

- 2 large eggs

- ½ cup Greek yogurt

- 1 tbsp honey

- 1 tbsp vanilla extract

- ½ cup fresh or frozen berries (for compote)

## Instructions

1. In a bowl, mix oat flour and baking powder.

2. In another bowl, whisk eggs, Greek yogurt, honey, and vanilla.

3. Combine the wet and dry ingredients until the batter is smooth.

4. Heat a non-stick skillet over medium heat and pour ¼ cup of batter for each pancake.

5. Cook until bubbles form on the surface, then flip and cook until golden.

6. For the compote, simmer berries in a small pot over low heat until they break down into a sauce.

7. Serve pancakes warm with berry compote on top.

## Golfer's Oatmeal Bowl

A sustaining meal that'll keep your energy levels steady throughout the morning. Steel-cut oats are my go-to. So good and keeps you feeling satisfied.

### Ingredients

- 1 cup steel-cut oats
- 3 cups water
- 1 apple, diced
- ¼ cup sliced almonds
- ½ tbsp cinnamon
- 1 tbsp maple syrup

### Instructions

1. Bring water to a boil in a saucepan.
2. Add oats and simmer on low for 20-25 minutes until oats are tender.
3. Stir in diced apple, almonds, and cinnamon in the last 5 minutes.
4. Serve hot, drizzled with maple syrup.

## Blueberry Almond Overnight Oats

### Ingredients

- ½ cup old-fashioned rolled oats

- ½ cup unsweetened almond milk (or your favorite milk)

- ½ cup fresh or frozen blueberries

- 1 tbsp almond butter

- 1 tbsp sliced almonds

- 1 tbsp chia seeds (optional)

- 1 tbsp honey or pure maple syrup (optional)

- A pinch of cinnamon (optional)

- A pinch of salt

### Instructions

1. In a container with a tight-fitting lid, combine the oats, almond milk, almond butter, and chia seeds (if using). Stir until well combined.

2. Mix in the blueberries, honey (if using), cinnamon, and a pinch of salt. Stir again.

3. Cover the container and refrigerate overnight (at least 6-8 hours).

4. In the morning, give it a quick stir. Add the sliced almonds on top for a crunchy finish.

5. Enjoy chilled or warm it up in the microwave if you prefer.

## Spinach and Feta Egg Muffins

These egg muffins are quick to make, portable, and packed with protein. They're great for early tee times because you can bake them the night before and grab a couple on your way out the door.

### Ingredients

- 6 eggs
- ½ cup spinach, chopped
- ¼ cup crumbled feta cheese
- Salt and pepper to taste
- Non-stick cooking spray

## Instructions

1. Preheat your oven to 350°F (175°C) and lightly coat a muffin tin with non-stick spray.

2. In a mixing bowl, whisk the eggs, then stir in the spinach, feta, salt, and pepper.

3. Pour the mixture into the muffin cups, filling each about three-quarters full.

4. Bake for 18-20 minutes or until the eggs are set and lightly golden.

5. Let them cool for a few minutes, then pop them out. Store extras in the fridge and reheat in the microwave the next morning.

Feel free to change up the ingredients. For example, add some chopped mushrooms, bell peppers, or onions.

## Veggie Omelet with Whole Grain Toast

### Ingredients

- 2-3 eggs or egg whites or tofu

- A handful of spinach

- Chopped bell peppers

- Diced tomatoes

- Sprinkle of cheese (optional)

- 1 slice of whole grain toast

- A small avocado

- Fresh fruit on the side (like an apple or orange)

### Instructions

1. Whisk the eggs in a bowl, then pour into a heated non-stick pan.

2. Add the spinach, bell peppers, and tomatoes. Cook until the eggs are set and the veggies are tender.

3. Sprinkle with a bit of cheese if you like.

4. While the omelet is cooking, toast the whole grain bread. Once it's done, top it with sliced avocado.

5. Plate the omelet and toast, and add some fresh fruit on the side for a well-rounded, nutrient-dense meal.

## Quinoa Breakfast Bowl

### Ingredients

- 1 cup cooked quinoa

- ½ cup low-fat Greek yogurt

- ½ cup mixed berries (strawberries, blueberries, raspberries)

- A handful of nuts (like almonds or walnuts)

- A drizzle of honey

- A sprinkle of chia seeds or flaxseeds

### Instructions

1. Cook the quinoa according to package instructions. Let it cool slightly.

2. In a bowl, layer the cooked quinoa, Greek yogurt, and mixed berries.

3. Top with a handful of nuts, a drizzle of honey, and a sprinkle of chia seeds or flaxseeds.

4. Mix everything together and enjoy a protein-packed, fiber-rich breakfast.

**Healthy Breakfast Muffin** (my favorite!)

**Ingredients**

- 1 ¼ cups whole wheat or all purpose flour

- 1 cup quick cooking oats

- 2 tsp baking soda

- ½ tsp ginger

- ½ tsp salt

- 2 tsp cinnamon

- 3 large eggs

- ¾ cup unsweetened apple sauce

- ⅓ cup olive oil

- ⅓ cup maple syrup

- 2 cups grated carrot

- 1 cup grated zucchini (make sure to squeeze out the water)

- ½ cup walnuts or pecans (optional)

- ½ cup cranberries (optional)

- 3 tbsp of ground flax or chia seeds

**Instructions**

1. Preheat oven to 375°F. Grease a muffin tin. Makes about 15 muffins.

2. In a medium bowl. Whisk together the flour, oats, baking soda, ginger, salt, and cinnamon.

3. In a larger bowl, whisk together the eggs, applesauce, oil, and maple syrup.

4. Add the dry ingredients to the wet and mix together. Do not overmix.

5. Fold in the carrots, zucchini, cranberries, walnuts/pecans, and ground flax/chia seeds.

6. Pour batter into the greased muffin tins. You can fill them to the top.

7. Bake for about 20 minutes and check to see if done. Internal temperature should reach 200°F.

## SNACKS TO SUSTAIN YOUR GAME

### Hole-in-One Hummus with Veggie Snacks

This homemade hummus is your secret weapon. Perfect for a mid-game refresh that's both nutritious and hydrating.

### Ingredients

- 1 can chickpeas, drained and rinsed

- 2 tbsp tahini

- Juice of 1 lemon

- 2 cloves garlic, minced

- Salt to taste

- Olive oil

- Assorted vegetable sticks (carrots, cucumber, bell peppers)

### Instructions

1. In a food processor, combine chickpeas, tahini, lemon juice, garlic, and a pinch of salt.

2. Process until smooth, adding olive oil as needed to achieve a creamy texture.

3. Serve with fresh vegetable sticks.

**No-Bake DIY Energy Balls**

**Ingredients**

- 1 cup old-fashioned rolled oats

- ½ cup natural peanut butter (or almond butter)

- 2-3 tbsp honey or pure maple syrup

- 2 tbsp ground flaxseed or chia seeds (optional)

- ¼ cup dried cranberries or chopped dates or chocolate chips (optional)

- A pinch of cinnamon (optional)

## Instructions

1. In a mixing bowl, combine the oats, peanut butter, and honey. Stir well with a spoon until the mixture starts to come together.

2. If using, add the ground flaxseed or chia seeds, dried fruit, and a pinch of cinnamon. Stir until everything is evenly mixed.

3. If the mixture seems too dry, add a little more nut butter or honey/maple syrup, and if it's too sticky, mix in a bit more oats.

4. Scoop out about a tbsp of the mixture and roll it between your palms to form a ball. Repeat with the remaining mixture.

5. Place the energy balls on a plate or baking sheet and refrigerate for at least 20 minutes so they can firm up.

6. Store them in an airtight container in the fridge for up to a week. They're great to grab before a morning

tee time or toss in your bag for an energy boost on the course.

## Fairway Trail Mix

A sweet and salty treat that tackles those mid-round hunger pangs and keeps your focus sharp.

### Ingredients

- ½ cup almonds

- ½ cup walnuts

- ⅓ cup pumpkin seeds

- ⅓ cup dried cherries (use any kind of dried food you would like)

- ⅓ cup dark chocolate chips

### Instructions

1. Simply mix all ingredients in a bowl.

2. Store in an airtight container and grab a handful whenever you need a quick energy boost.

**Easy Roasted Chickpeas**

A crunchy protein-packed snack.

**Instructions**

- 1 can (15 oz) chickpeas, drained and rinsed

- 1 tbsp olive oil

- ½ tbsp salt

- ½ tsp smoked paprika (or your favorite spice blend)

- A pinch of black pepper

**Instructions**

1. Preheat your oven to 400°F (200°C).

2. Pat the chickpeas dry with a clean kitchen towel or paper towel. The drier they are, the crispier they'll get.

3. Spread the chickpeas on a baking sheet. Drizzle with olive oil, then sprinkle with salt, smoked paprika, and black pepper. Gently toss to coat.

4. Roast for about 20-30 minutes, shaking the pan halfway through, until the chickpeas are crispy on the outside.

5. Let them cool for a few minutes before snacking. Store any leftovers in an airtight container. However, they're best eaten the same day for maximum crunch.

## DINNER DELIGHTS

### The 19th Hole Stir Fry

After a long day on the course, come home to a hearty stir-fry. A great way to replenish your body and comfort your soul.

(Serves 2-4 people depending on portion size)

### Ingredients

- 2 chicken breasts, thinly sliced

- 2 cups broccoli florets

- 1 bell pepper, sliced

- 1 cup snap peas

- 2 cloves garlic, minced

- 1 tbsp fresh ginger, minced

- 2 tbsp soy sauce

- 1 tbsp olive oil

- Cooked brown rice for serving

**Instructions**

1. Heat olive oil in a large skillet over medium-high heat.

2. Add garlic and ginger, and sauté for 30 seconds.

3. Add chicken and stir-fry until nearly cooked through.

4. Add broccoli, bell pepper, and snap peas, cooking until vegetables are tender.

5. Stir in soy sauce and cook for an additional minute.

6. Serve hot over brown rice.

## Champion's Chili

It's perfect for refueling after a day of driving and putting.

### Ingredients

- 1 lb ground turkey (Could use vegan ground beef or tofu)
- 1 can kidney beans, drained
- 1 can diced tomatoes
- 1 onion, chopped
- 2 cloves garlic, minced
- 1 tbsp chili powder
- 1 tsp cumin
- Salt and pepper to taste
- Olive oil

### Instructions

1. Heat a large pot over medium heat and add a splash of olive oil.

2. Add onion and garlic, sauté until soft.

3. Add ground turkey, break it up with a spoon, and cook until browned.

4. Stir in tomatoes, beans, chili powder, and cumin.

5. Simmer for at least 30 minutes, stirring occasionally.

6. Season with salt and pepper to taste and serve.

**Grilled Salmon with Quinoa Salad**

This dinner packs in omega-3s for brain health and protein for muscle recovery, making it the perfect way to end your active day.

**Ingredients**

- 4 salmon fillets

- 1 cup quinoa

- 2 cups water

- 2 cups arugula

- 1 avocado, diced

- ½ cup pomegranate seeds

- Juice of 1 lemon

- Olive oil

- Salt and pepper

**Instructions**

1. Rinse quinoa under cold water.

2. In a saucepan, bring water to a boil, add quinoa, reduce to a simmer, cover, and cook for 15 minutes.

3. Season salmon fillets with salt and pepper and grill over medium heat, about 4 minutes per side.

4. Fluff quinoa with a fork, then mix in arugula, avocado, and pomegranate seeds.

5. Dress the salad with lemon juice and a drizzle of olive oil.

6. Serve the grilled salmon over the quinoa salad.

## The Best Veggie Burger

These are yummy and perfect for refueling after a long day on the course. Add some fresh veggies or a side salad, and you've got a well-rounded meal that supports recovery.

## Ingredients

- 1 can (15 oz) (425 grams) chickpeas
- ½ red onion finely diced
- 1 zucchini, grated
- 1 cup (70 grams) mushrooms, diced
- 3 tbsp cilantro, finely chopped
- 3 tbsp red wine vinegar
- 1 tbsp sriracha
- 2 tbsp tahini
- 1 tsp cumin
- ½ tsp garlic powder
- 1-2 tsp black pepper

- 1 tbsp ground flaxseed

- ½ tsp sea salt

- 1 cup (80 grams) quick oats (gluten-free)

- 2 tbsp extra virgin olive oil

- Extra virgin olive oil (for sautéing)

**Instructions**

1. Drain and rinse the chickpeas. Then, in a large bowl, mash them with a fork.

2. Add the remainder of the ingredients and mix well.

3. Form into 6-8 patties.

4. Place in the refrigerator for 10-15 minutes to give the patties time to become firm.

5. Heat about 1 tbsp olive oil in a skillet over medium heat. When hot, place the patties in the skillet and sauté for 4-6 minutes per side.

From breakfast bites to end-of-day dinners, the recipes here are all about nourishing both your body and your mind.

Think of good food as another club in your bag … one that can help you focus, stay energized, and swing with ease.

Eat well, play well, and maybe your next meal will lead you straight to a hole-in-one!

# Hole 15

# Course Corrections

# Nutrition Strategies for Common Golf Challenges

Golf is a very humbling game that can be unpredictable. One moment, you're playing like you can do nothing wrong, and the next moment, you're struggling to keep the ball in play.

Or, you have a hot front nine and think you're on your way to your best game ever. Only to have a back nine that falls apart.

And you're wondering, "What the heck happened!?"

Lost my swing? The wind picked up? It's too hot? Etc.

The biggest reason for this could be loss of mental focus and energy. Which, in turn, could be caused by not fueling your body properly.

And, as you now know, your nutrition plays a significant role.

In this chapter, we'll explore common challenges you may encounter on the course and how proper nutrition can help you overcome them.

Challenges such as fatigue, loss of focus, and those unpleasant nerves fluttering around in your stomach as you get ready to hit a key shot!

**Fatigue Fighters**

Fatigue is a common concern for many golfers. You start your game feeling great, energized, and focused but somewhere on the back nine, your energy drops, and so does your game.

This mostly happens because of depleted energy stores and dehydration.

The strategy to help keep your energy up isn't just about what and when you eat but also about when and how you hydrate.

Your day should start with a solid breakfast that balances complex carbs with proteins: think a hearty oatmeal topped with nuts or a smoothie packed with fruits, Greek yogurt, and a scoop of protein powder.

During the round, it's important that you snack smartly. An energy bar, banana, handful of mixed nuts, or a peanut butter sandwich can be your best friends, providing a steady release of energy to keep those swings sharp till the last putt.

For an example of a guideline of when and what to eat, check out Hole 9.

Hydrate, hydrate, hydrate. The best thing you can do for yourself when it comes to hydration is to hydrate properly EVERY day and not just when you know you are going to golf.

However, if your hydration is not up to par, then make sure to hydrate well a day before your game. Pre-hydration helps maintain stamina and prevent the onset of fatigue.

On the day, drink water mixed with electrolytes before starting, and keep sipping every few holes. Electrolytes help with fluid balance and muscle function, preventing cramps and fatigue.

You can also drink coconut water.

**Staying Sharp**

Losing focus can quietly sabotage your score. To keep your mind sharp, fuel up with foods rich in omega-3 fatty acids and antioxidants.

Think a salmon sandwich on whole grain bread, a berry-filled salad with walnuts, bell peppers with hummus, or a handful of nuts.

These are great snacks that will boost your brain health, improve concentration, and help with decision-making.

And don't forget hydration. It's essential! Dehydration can dull your focus, so drink water regularly and consider coconut water or electrolyte drinks to stay properly hydrated throughout your round.

**Easing Nerves and Stress**

Lastly, let's talk about nerves.

Feeling jittery can really throw off your game, making even the easiest shots feel daunting.

Try to incorporate magnesium-rich foods into your diet. Magnesium has natural calming properties that can help soothe your nerves.

Snack on nuts and seeds, or sip a smoothie with spinach and yogurt before your game to harness these benefits.

Steady sugar levels mean steady nerves.

Therefore, avoid high-sugar foods that can spike and crash your energy and mood. Opt for slow-digesting carbs like oats, whole wheat bread, sweet potatoes, quinoa, or roasted chickpeas, which provide long-lasting energy and keep those butterflies under control.

The gut-brain connection plays an important role in how stress affects the body. Include probiotic-rich foods like yogurt, kefir, kimchi, sauerkraut, or pickles (fermented in brine) in your diet to help support gut health, which in turn can help manage stress and improve overall mood.

When adding probiotics to your diet, it's also important to include prebiotic foods like fiber-rich vegetables and whole grains. These help fuel the growth of beneficial bacteria in your gut, ensuring that the probiotics can thrive and do their job effectively.

And don't forget hydration. Good hydration helps with focus and endurance, keeping you mentally and physically sharp.

There is a recurring theme throughout the challenges.

Eat smart and hydrate!

Each meal, snack, and drink choice becomes part of your strategy to maintain energy, focus, and calmness, making nutrition a powerful tool to have in your golf bag.

When your energy and focus are good, you will be able to play more consistently. Something we all strive for!

Remember, in golf, as in nutrition, it's all about making the right choices at the right time.

As we wrap up managing the challenges you face on the course, it's time to shift gears and put everything we've discussed into action.

At the next hole, we'll share tips on how to put it all together so that it works for you.

# Hole 16

# Putting It All Together

Hopefully, you have picked up some great tips to help you get an edge on your game. This next section is to help you pull together the strategies you have learned so far into a solid game plan.

Think of this as creating your own nutrition playbook, designed to keep your energy strong and mind focused from the first tee to the 18th green.

### Craft Your Custom Nutrition Playbook

Your nutrition plan should be as unique as your golf game. Start by considering your specific dietary needs, preferences, and goals.

- Do you need a quick energy boost before the game?

- Are you aiming for steady energy throughout?

- Are there any dietary restrictions, like managing diabetes or gluten intolerance?

Make a note of these as your playbook's foundation.

Then, map out a typical game day. Schedule your meals and snacks around your tee time. If you have an early morning game, ensure your breakfast is filling but not heavy, and pack mid-game snacks like a banana or a handful of nuts. The goal is to avoid the dreaded mid-round slump, so timing your intake is just as important as what you eat.

Check out Hole 9, which provides an example of what your schedule could look like.

Remember, the goal is to prevent the mid-round slump, so timing your intake is as crucial as what you eat.

At the end of this section, there is a Golfer's Daily Nutrition Journal that you can use to help you monitor your nutrition and hydration intake and how you are feeling in terms of energy and focus.

If you are not strategic about how you fuel up and find yourself having energy slumps during your round, then the Nutrition Journal could work for you.

**Meal Prep Like a Pro**

Meal prepping is more than just a time-saver; it's about making sure you're ready for game time without scrambling around in the kitchen or relying on the snack shack's less-than-healthy options.

Set aside some time over the weekend or on a weekday or night (whatever works for you) to plan and prepare your meals.

- Cook grains like rice or quinoa in bulk,

- Chop veggies and portion them out into containers for easy grab-and-go.

- Make extra chicken, beef, tofu, etc, at dinner and use it for sandwiches the next day.

- Make sure to have bananas and apples on hand to grab and go.

- Prep your snacks, such as trail mix or energy balls

- Boil a few hard-boiled eggs

- Have electrolytes ready to go or coconut water

Being prepared is key to staying on track with your nutrition throughout the round.

### Keep Your Nutrition Game on Par

Try to be consistent with your nutrition and adaptable.

Start by sticking to the basics of your plan, but be ready to adapt based on how you feel each day. If you find certain foods don't sit well during a game, switch them out.

Listen to your body … it's the best coach you'll ever have.

Also, keep your motivation high by celebrating small victories. Made it through a whole round without hitting the snack bar? That's a win.

Hydrated well and felt great after the game? Another win.

Lastly, remember that nutrition is just one part of your golfing experience. Combine what you've learned here with good physical training, adequate sleep, and mental preparation.

This holistic approach will not only improve your game but enhance your overall health and enjoyment of the sport.

And there you have it! Remember, every meal is an opportunity to fuel your body optimally; every snack is a chance to fine-tune your energy levels.

With this playbook, you're set not just to play but to play at your peak.

Creating a daily food journal tailored for golfers can be a great way to keep track of nutrition and its impact on performance. Here's a template you might find useful:

**Golfer's Daily Nutrition Journal**

The following journal will not only help you monitor what you eat and drink but also how your body responds to different foods and timings, and dietary needs.

## Golfer's Daily Nutrition Journal

**Date:**_____

**Tee Time:** _____

---

## Personal Preferences & Goals

**Dietary Restrictions/Allergies:** _____

**Goal Focus for Today:** _____ (e.g., muscle recovery, hydration, energy maintenance)

---

## Morning (Pre-Game)

## Breakfast:

- What did you eat? _____
- Time eaten: _____
- Portion size: _____

## Hydration:

- Hydration goal for today (oz): _____

- Water intake (oz): _____

- Did you add any electrolytes? _____

---

## On-Course Snacks

## Snack #1 (Holes 1-6):

- What did you eat? _____

- Portion size: _____

- Energy level (1-10): _____

- Mental Focus (1-10): _____

## Snack #2 (Holes 7-12):

- What did you eat? _____

- Portion size: _____

- Energy level (1-10): _____

- Mental Focus (1-10): _____

## Snack #3 (Holes 13-18):

- What did you eat? _____
- Portion size: _____
- Energy level (1-10): _____
- Mental Focus (1-10): _____

---

## Post-Round Recovery

## Post-Game Meal/Snack:

- What did you eat after your round? _____
- Portion size: _____
- Energy level (1-10): _____

## Post Round Hydration:

- Post-round hydration goal (oz): _____

- Water intake (oz): _____

- Electrolyte drinks: _____

## Daily Reflections:

- Did you meet your goals?

  _____

- Overall Hydration Assessment:

  _____

- Mood and Energy:

  _____

- Suggestions for Tomorrow: (adjustments in timing, type of food, hydration strategy, etc.)

  _____

# Hole 17

# Progress Over Perfection

A few important things to remember as you work on improving your nutrition for better golf.

## Progress Over Perfection

Perfection isn't the goal … and it's not realistic. If the thought of implementing all that you read seems overwhelming, then start by setting small, achievable goals. The process of forming new habits is just as important as the end result.

For example, if hydration is your focus, aim to drink more water during your round. If you don't hit your exact target but you do drink more than usual, that's still a win! The next time you golf, try to drink just a little bit more. Every step counts and will build momentum.

And, if eating healthier snacks is your goal and you find that you only ate 2 of your 3 or 4 snacks, which is better than you usually do, that's still a win! Just keep on working on it.

Building habits takes time and effort. And, if you are not perfect, no worries. Don't be hard on yourself! There is no such thing as perfection. Just keep practicing, and before you know it, your new habit(s) will become second nature.

For some of you, mastering hydration might be a big enough goal to begin with. Once you feel confident in that, you can gradually focus on other aspects, like improving your snacks or planning your meals.

It's all about making steady progress, not achieving perfection. Know that small changes will lead to big results over time.

**Tame Your Inner Critic**

When self-doubt creeps in, especially when it comes to making change, it's easy to believe negative thoughts like I'll never stick to this plan" or "I'm not disciplined enough."

Take a moment and ask yourself, "Is this really true?" The answer is often no. The reason for those thoughts usually comes from fear.

To help with the fear, start small. Remember, Progress over Perfection. Small wins add up over time, and the effort you put into nourishing your body will lead to more energy and focus which leads to better golf.

Self-doubt also grows when we compare ourselves to others, but your journey is unique. Each healthier choice you make, whether it's staying hydrated or choosing better snacks, brings you closer to your goal.

Reframe your negative thoughts with empowering affirmations such as "I'm capable of making better choices." or "Mistakes are part of the learning process, not failures."

With time and practice, you'll find that you feel more confident. You'll begin to feel better both on and off the course.

## Celebrate Small Wins

When you celebrate small wins, you build confidence and momentum. Too often, we focus on the big picture and not the smaller steps that we take to get there.

But each small success … even if it's 2 cups more of water, one healthy snack added to your day, or a good breakfast … deserves recognition.

These small wins are proof of your progress and commitment. By celebrating them, you reinforce positive behaviors and create a sense of accomplishment, which motivates you to keep going.

Why not write down your wins. This will help you to stay focused and appreciate how far you have come!

Or share your wins with a coach, family, or friends. Their support will provide positive reinforcement and motivation, which will help keep you on track.

# Hole 18

# From Tee to Beyond

It should be clear now that your golf game is shaped not just by your swing but by what you eat and drink.

In this section, we'll take a look at how the right nutrition not only powers your game but also supports long-term vitality, ensuring you're playing your best both now and for years to come.

## How the Right Meals Make More Pars and Birdies

There's a direct link between what's on your plate and what's on your scorecard. Meals that are rich in lean proteins, whole grains, healthy fats, and fresh vegetables can boost your concentration and your stamina, reducing fatigue as you approach the last few holes.

Imagine standing on the 16th tee, feeling just as good as you did on the first. That's the power of proper nutrition.

Plus, there's a psychological boost of knowing you're fueling your body well. So, when you step onto the green, confident in your body's readiness, you experience a more relaxed, focused state of mind, helping you make those clutch putts.

## Hydration: Your Best Friend On and Off the Course

We have talked a lot about hydration, and for good reason, as it's your best friend in both golf and life.

Water helps maintain your concentration, energy, and overall health. Just like a great caddie, it's always there for you, supporting your body through the ups and downs of the game.

It helps:

- Regulate body temperature.

- Lubricates joints.

- Deliver nutrients to your cells.

- Increase endurance.

- Maintain focus.

- Improve your mood.

All important for your golf game! Staying hydrated also helps prevent long-term health issues like kidney stones, constipation, headaches, and urinary tract infections.

Whether it's during a round or as part of your daily routine, water is key to playing your best and living your best life.

**Adjusting Your Dietary Strategy for Steady Improvement**

Just as you may tweak your stance or grip to improve your swing, your diet may need to be adjusted too. As you age, your body's needs can change. Therefore, your nutrition should be adjusted to meet its needs.

Every time you are playing, pay attention to how your body responds.

Did you eat enough? If you are feeling tired, maybe you need to adjust your snacks for more energy, or maybe you need to eat a balanced, nutrient-dense meal post-game to recharge.

Did you drink enough? If you are experiencing a loss of focus, have no energy, or have a headache, maybe you need to adjust your water and electrolyte intake.

It might be a good idea for you to hydrate well post-game and plan to increase your water intake on the course for the following game. Especially if it's hot out.

There's no one-size-fits-all approach in golf or nutrition, so tailor your food choices to your body's needs and your game's demands.

**Consistency is Key**

If you're thinking that this will require a big cleanup of your pantry and fridge, let me stop you right there.

This isn't about doing a complete lifestyle change overnight. That would only set you up for failure.

Think of it more like improving your golf swing. Small, consistent changes, like adding a fruit or veggie to every meal or swapping out that afternoon chocolate bar for a handful of nuts, will lead to big wins over time.

It's about being consistent and making progress.

It's not about eliminating treats but making sure they don't dominate your diet.

Yes, you can still enjoy your post-round beer/wine and burgers.

It's all about finding the sweet spot where enjoyment and health meet.

Just like balance is key in golf, it's also key in eating. And when you find that balance, you create a sustainable eating pattern that supports your game and overall health.

**Linking Golf Nutrition to Lifelong Vitality**

Fact: what we put in our bodies affects our performance on the course.

But, the benefits of smart nutrition extend far beyond the golf course. Whether you're swinging clubs or chasing grandkids, a diet rich in nutrients supports your energy levels, brain function, and overall well-being.

Just like choosing the right club for your shot, choosing the right foods sets you up for success ... on the course and in life.

## The Long Game: How Nutrition Protects Your Health

Think of your body as a well-maintained golf bag. If you fill it with the right equipment, you'll be ready for any challenge.

Just as you wouldn't use broken clubs, don't fuel your body with processed foods. Choosing whole, nutrient-dense foods like fruits, vegetables, lean proteins, healthy fats, and whole grains is like selecting your best clubs for the shot.

Another bonus of eating well is that these foods help prevent chronic diseases like diabetes, heart disease, and high blood pressure, allowing you to play strong for years to come.

By investing in your nutrition, you're setting yourself up for long-term health ... both on and off the course.

## In Closing

Nutrition isn't a one-time fix ... it's a lifelong commitment to fueling your body, improving your performance, and enhancing your well-being.

And, just like golf, it's a continuous process of learning, adjusting, and refining.

With every nutritious meal, think of it as adding yards to your drive, precision to your shots, and years to your life. Now, that's what I call playing the long game.

## About The Author

Anita is a holistic nutrition coach and lifelong athlete dedicated to helping people live a life of quality and vitality. With a passion for fueling smarter, she's created and successfully delivered holistic nutrition programs that help clients build sustainable habits.

And, as a three-time world champion in dragon boating, provincial golf title holder, and figure competitor, Anita knows what it takes to stay strong under pressure and understands how nutrition can positively impact performance.

When she noticed too many golfers crashing on the back nine — fueled by candy bars, skipped meals, and dehydration — The Golfer's Nutrition Caddy was born: a practical, no-nonsense guide to staying strong, focused and energized from the first tee to the final putt.

While nutrition plays a starring role in Anita's playbook, she knows it's just one part of the performance puzzle. She champions a whole-person approach — quality sleep, flexibility and mobility exercises, focused practice, and a positive mindset all help golfers feel their best so they can play their best.

Anita's experience as both an athlete and a coach has shaped her real-world, down-to-earth style. She's helped countless clients shift their health habits through personalized, sustainable strategies — no gimmicks, no guilt, just steady progress.

The best part? The energy, confidence, and focus you gain on the course will spill over into your life off the course, too — helping you feel more vibrant and in control no matter where you are.

Whether you're chasing par or just trying to stay focused on the back nine, Anita's here to help you fuel with confidence — and maybe even shave off a few strokes, one smart snack at a time.

# Acknowledgement

Writing this book has been an incredible journey, and I couldn't have done it without the support, encouragement, and wisdom of so many wonderful people.

A heartfelt thank you to **Norma**, whose keen eye and thoughtful feedback were invaluable in the reading and editing process. Your encouragement and support made all the difference.

I'm incredibly grateful to **Nancy**, who was always there when uncertainty crept in. Whether it was refining the wording, helping with the cover, or simply talking things through, her insight and encouragement were invaluable. Your support throughout this journey meant so much — thank you.

To **MC**, always a pro on and off the course, thank you for your support and belief in this project. Knowing that someone so immersed in the game found value in these pages was an incredible boost.

To **Gio**, whose quiet support and thoughtful insights were truly appreciated — thank you.

To my **golfing buddies**, who have been cheering me on and eagerly awaiting this book, your support, encouragement, and shared love of the game mean more than you know. I hope this book serves you well both on and off the course!

To the **wonderful women at my course**, whose warmth, camaraderie, and love for the game have made every season even more enjoyable. Playing with you has been an absolute joy, and I'm grateful for the fun, laughter, and great rounds we've shared.

To my **family**, whose steady support and patience have meant so much — I appreciate you more than words can say.

To my **mentors**, fellow wellness professionals, and those who have shared their wisdom with me over the years — thank you for shaping my understanding and deepening my passion for this work.

A sincere thank you to **KDP Publishers** for bringing this book to life and for your patience in navigating my revisions and changes along the way.

And finally, to **you**, the reader — thank you for picking up this book, for trusting me to guide you, and for believing that a stronger, healthier, more vibrant game (and life!) is within reach. I hope this book serves as a valuable guide on and off the course.

With gratitude,

**Anita**

PS: Any questions or comments, feel free to email me at AnitaDuwel@live.com